The 4-Week
Endometriosis
Diet Plan

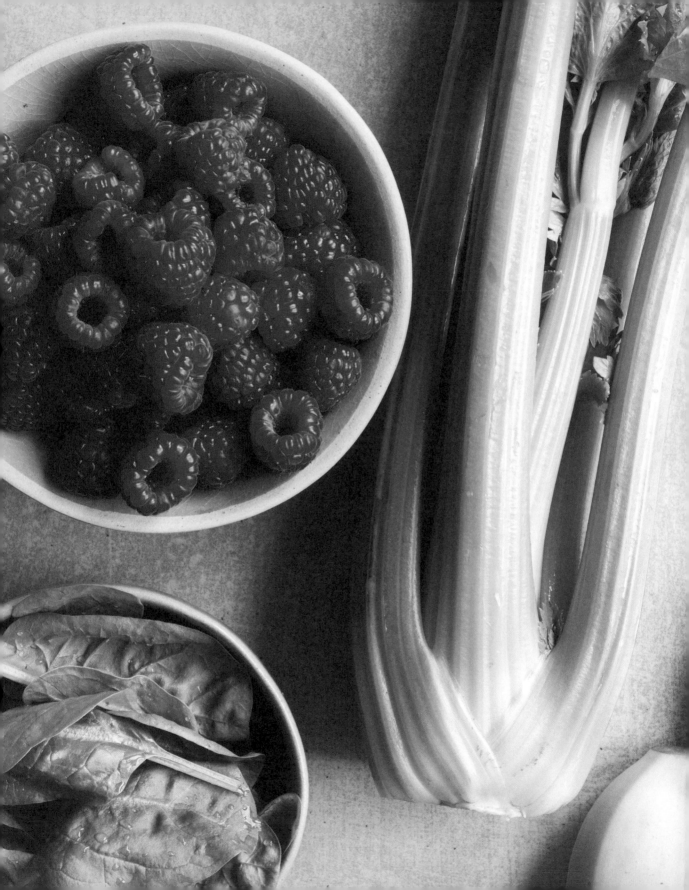

The *The* 4-Week *Endometriosis* Diet Plan

75 **Healing Recipes** to Relieve Symptoms *and* Regain Control of Your Life

by Katie Edmonds, NTC

Foreword by **Aviva Romm, MD**

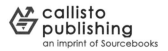

callisto
publishing
an imprint of Sourcebooks

Copyright © 2019 by Callisto Publishing LLC

Cover and internal design © 2019 by Callisto Publishing LLC

Photography © Becky Staynor, cover, p.xii, 12, 24, 34, 42, 56, 58, 70, 90, 102, 114, 126, 138;
Nadine Greeff, p.ii, 32; Darren Muir, p.vi; Hélène Dujardin, p.xiv.

Food styling by Kathleen Phillips, cover, p.xii, 12, 24, 34, 42, 56, 58, 70, 90, 102, 114, 126, 138.

Illustrations used under license from Shutterstock.com.

Interior and Cover Designer: Stephanie Mautone

Art Producer: Sara Feinstein

Editor: Marjorie DeWitt

Production Manager: Holly Haydash

Production Editors: Melissa Edeburn and Erum Khan

Published by Callisto Publishing LLC C/O Sourcebooks LLC
P.O. Box 4410, Naperville, Illinois 60567-4410
(630) 961-3900
callistopublishing.com

Printed and Bound In China
OGP 16

Dedication

Dedicated to my amazing family, my miracle son, and every woman who's ever suffered with endometriosis.

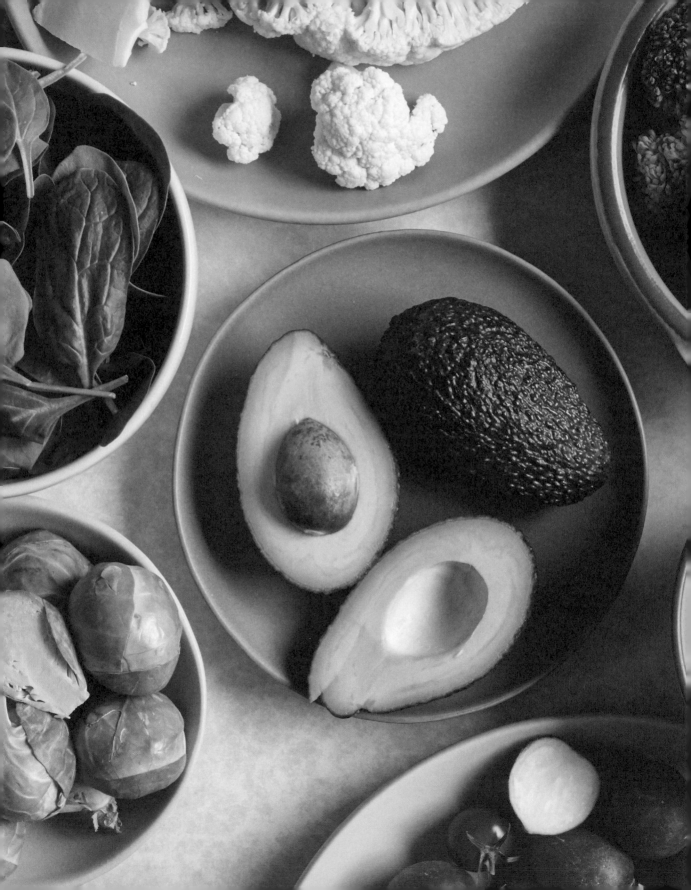

CONTENTS

FOREWORD

Endometriosis is a diagnosis an increasing number of women are receiving each year. From teens with debilitating pain on their *first* period, to much-too-young women facing fertility challenges, and even women well into their forties still battling pelvic pain, digestive symptoms, and more, endometriosis seems to know no boundaries. Although awareness is slowly increasing, it takes an average of nearly 10 years to get a proper diagnosis, and even with one, there is still an alarmingly inadequate level of care for many of these women who are living with chronic pain. As a Yale-trained MD, midwife, herbalist, mother, and leading expert in women's health, I am saddened to know how many women are left without hope, and how few options most sufferers feel they have in reclaiming their health.

That's why I'm excited about the publication of *The 4-Week Endometriosis Diet Plan*. More than just recipes, this book contains information that allows women from all walks of life to understand the enormous complexity of endometriosis—a condition with underlying causes that span far beyond the pelvis—as dozens of scientific articles help us understand—and thus a condition that requires a holistic approach to healing of both symptoms *and* causes.

Within these pages I am thrilled to see often-missing information that can help you shift beyond the current limited drugs-and-surgery paradigm with a fresh approach. You'll be inspired by the list of nourishing foods that should be at the center of your healing plan—tons of vegetables, healthy oils, and pastured or 100 percent grass-fed meats—all served with a big side of essential information on movement, stress reduction, and alternative therapies to take with you on your unique endo-healing journey.

This book is a guide to help women through the seemingly disconnected set of symptoms associated with endometriosis, and it offers an integrative approach every woman with endometriosis can apply *now*. Perhaps what's especially important about this book is that it's written by a woman who understands what endometriosis means in real life. As a former endometriosis sufferer, Katie helps you apply the tools in her book to address the struggles faced by women with endometriosis every day.

As anyone who has used a Band-Aid approach to treating endometriosis knows, one method alone is rarely successful at preserving fertility and quality of life—or at maintaining hope. To address this condition, we need a smart, integrative framework and a multitude of healing modalities with a nourishing approach at the forefront. You will find these tools in this book.

Wishing you a healing journey.

Aviva Romm, MD

Author of The Adrenal Thyroid Revolution *and the forthcoming*
The HormonEcology Solution *(Harper One, 2020)*

INTRODUCTION

When I was diagnosed with endometriosis nearly a decade ago, I went home and collapsed in tears. The pain had been so intense, so crippling, I assumed it was cancer. Many tests later, only one possibility remained: endometriosis. I couldn't believe it, since I naively thought endo was "just" painful periods. My pain was all the time, and to be told at 24 years old that your crippling pain has no cure; that you can only treat the symptoms with birth control, pain killers, and surgeries; and that children may not be in your future was, to me, so much worse than cancer.

Fast forward 10 years and I'm healthier than I was before my diagnosis and subsequent downward spiral from pharmaceuticals and stress. I'm even healthier than before onset of my pre-endo health issues. Now I have natural energy for the first time in decades, my hormonal roller coaster is a thing of the past, my endometriosis is in full remission, and after two years of infertility I have a very healthy baby.

How did my health improve so dramatically? Diet and lifestyle. It was only when I stopped fearfully restricting foods and instead embraced nutrients, stopped stressing and learned to chill out, and improved my poor gut health that I was able to thrive. I now help clients from all over the world heal anew by addressing the myriad health issues *contributing to* endo rather than addressing endo symptoms. Through this approach I've seen many women reclaim their hopes, their fertility, and their lives.

If you're unsure how diet and lifestyle changes can affect some misplaced tissue in your pelvis, I can totally relate. When I was first diagnosed, my now-husband told me to look into diet. I laughed—not kidding—because why would what I put in my mouth have anything to do with my lady parts? Well, after a little sleuthing I found out he might be right—and today science is right there with him. We now have mounting research connecting the onset and severity of endometriosis with malnutrition, stress, pathogenic bacterial overgrowth in the gut (called dysbiosis), immune dysfunction, hormone imbalances, and endocrine-disrupting chemicals in our environment. It's when we view endo from this perspective that it becomes clear how holistic approaches can reduce the pain in your pelvis. Indeed, it's the only way you can truly address endo issues. There's no pill or surgery that can substitute for these approaches.

That said, diet or lifestyle alone is no magic pill for every endo sufferer. Endo is a complex disease that may require a combination of both conventional and alternative approaches tailored to each person. However, I still believe the approaches you'll find in this book are foundational for healing no matter who you are. Here, you'll find important nutritional information to better understand which foods are affecting you and why, how lifestyle changes can dramatically increase your quality of life, and clear instructions for a one-month couch-to-kitchen plan that will give you the motivation to tackle whole-foods cooking once and for all.

No one ever told me that with the correct approach I could resolve my endo and reclaim my life—I didn't even know it was a possibility. There may be no cure for endo, but we can change our habits to heal our bodies enough to live normal lives. Even if you can't achieve full remission, what if you could achieve 75 percent or even 50 percent remission? That's half the pain, half the fatigue, half the sadness. Sounds pretty good to me. That is the hope I wish to convey throughout this book. Plus, isn't life a lot more fun when you eat well and laugh often? Of course it is!

Welcome to the journey.

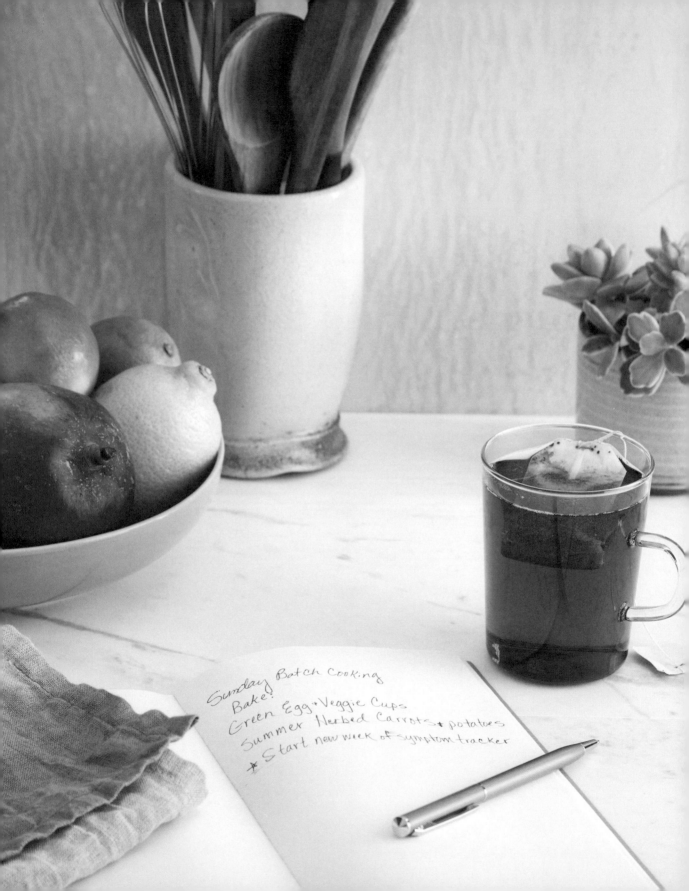

Sunday Batch Cooking
Bake!
Green Egg + Veggie Cups
Summer Herbed Carrots + potatoes
* Start new week of symptom tracker

PART I

The Endometriosis Guide

Endometriosis is a deceivingly complex disorder that, although common, is still often misunderstood. To choose your best path for healing, you need to know exactly what it is and how it affects your body. My goal is to help you do that. By better understanding your disease, you'll be better able to make the right decisions with your health care providers about which treatment plan is best and which additional holistic options may be beneficial for you.

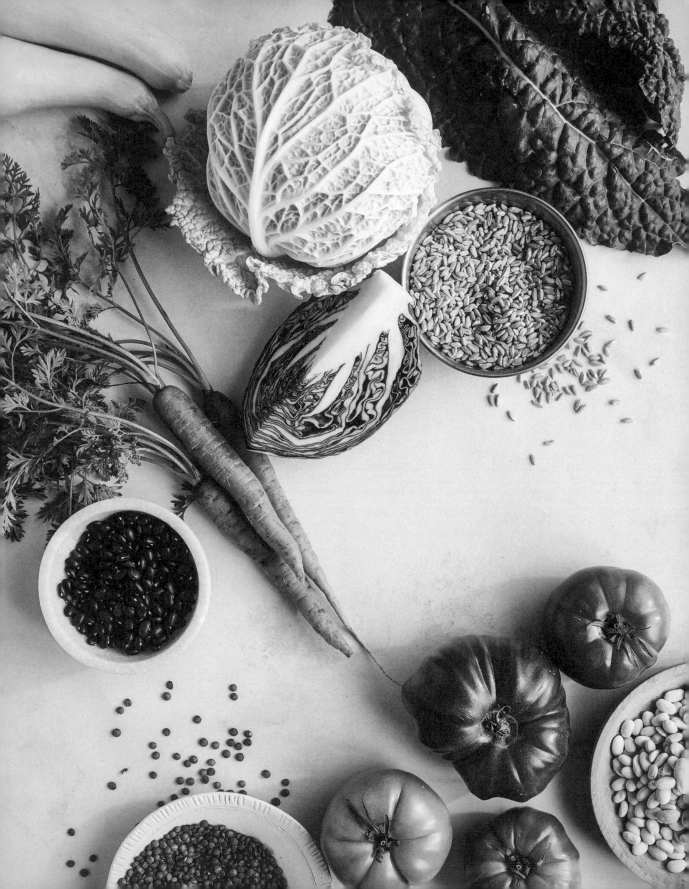

CHAPTER 1

Understanding Endometriosis

Endometriosis is a complex and debilitating disease affecting 1 in 10 women. Although the main symptoms are often related to the female reproductive system, endo is a full-body issue involving the immune, hormonal, and digestive systems. Approaching endo from a holistic perspective is beneficial for you to feel your best. By learning everything you can about your disease and how it affects your own body, you're already on the right path.

WHAT IS ENDOMETRIOSIS?

In the simplest terms, endometriosis is the painful condition in which tissue similar to the endometrium tissue that lines the uterus grows outside of the uterus. This endometriosis tissue grows mainly in the pelvic cavity, but it can also migrate to the digestive organs, diaphragm, and beyond. In its sister disease, adenomyosis, the tissue grows within the uterine wall. During every menstrual cycle, the lining grows and sheds, as a normal endometrium would, but because it can't escape the uterus as it should during a woman's menses, it instead sheds internally with no escape route. Now blood is freely flowing within the pelvic cavity where it should never be, leading to pelvic pain, inflammation, scar tissue, and, if left unchecked, damage to, or adhesion between, organs.

There are numerous theories about how endometriosis develops. One theory is that the misplaced endometrium lining may be abnormally placed before birth. Other theories are that endometriosis may develop through retrograde menstruation or that it may be the result of immunological issues or of toxin exposure. It may develop in multiple ways; research continues.

Endo has telltale signs, but only exploratory laparoscopic surgery can diagnose the disease and its stage, from stage I (least advanced) to stage IV (most advanced). Interestingly, level of pain does not seem to correlate with stage. You can have crippling pain with stage I and no pain at all with stage IV.

Women experiencing symptoms can wait years for a definitive diagnosis, leading to increased and unnecessary suffering. That suffering is why continued awareness is so important, why we must repeat "painful periods are not normal," and why widespread education about all the associated symptoms is a must. If we want to protect the fertility, bodies, hopes, and dreams of women everywhere, early diagnosis is key.

SYSTEMIC ISSUES

Symptoms of endo are often related to menstrual cycles, but we now know that endo is so much more than a "woman's condition." It's also an inflammatory, immunological, malnutritional, epigenetic/genetic, and gut-associated issue. Truly, endometriosis is a systemic issue reaching far beyond your pelvic cavity.

ENDO AS A HORMONAL DISEASE

The current dialogue suggests that we all are making way too much estrogen, but the answer to endo is not as straightforward as that. The real issue is estrogen dominance: too much estrogen in comparison to progesterone levels. The large amount of estrogen-mimicking chemicals in our everyday environment, as well as the fact that the endo lesions themselves are slightly progesterone-resistant, further damages our hormonal imbalance. All these factors combine to create an overly estrogenic state within the pelvis that constantly fuels more endo growth.

ENDO AS AN IMMUNE AND INFLAMMATORY ISSUE

Endometriosis is an autoimmune-related disease, which means that your immune system isn't working as it should. Both the innate and the adaptive immune systems aren't functioning correctly in the pelvic cavity, and this is *partly* responsible for both increased inflammation and reduced anti-inflammatory activities. This is why regulating the immune system is crucial to bringing down systemic levels of inflammation.

ENDO AS A GUT ISSUE

Like virtually all autoimmune and related disorders, endo appears to be an issue with the gut. Increased gut permeability, commonly known as leaky gut, is a condition in which the lining of your intestinal tract breaks down enough to allow toxins, bacteria, and food particles to "leak" through into the bloodstream. Dysbiosis is an imbalance within your gut microbiome or the microorganisms that live in your gut. Science is beginning to uncover just how much these issues may be playing a role in endo: Those who suffer have been shown to have gut microbiomes that are significantly altered for the worse. A 2016 study published in the *American Journal of Obstetrics and Gynecology* hypothesized that "gut microbiota may be involved crucially in the onset and progression of endometriosis," while a 2019 study in *Scientific Reports* discusses "whether dysbiosis leads to endometriosis or endometriosis leads to dysbiosis."

We also now know that the toxic byproduct of pathogenic bacteria from your gut—LPS, or lipopolysaccharide—directly stimulates endo implants to grow lesions and increase inflammation in the pelvic cavity. In fact, LPS was found to be four to six times higher in the menstrual blood of women with endo, with some varieties even colonizing the endo lesions themselves. How is the LPS getting to your pelvis? We could postulate that it's due to leaky gut, which is why healing and sealing the gut—and addressing that endo-belly—becomes a pivotal piece in reducing inflammation.

ENDO AS A MALNUTRITIONAL ISSUE

There is a definite link between endometriosis and malnutrition. Research shows nutrient deficiency may directly contribute to the development of endometriosis. Further studies show us endo-gals are either deficient in or could greatly benefit from increased amounts of vitamins A, C, D, and E, zinc, omega-3s, and selenium. This could be because we're either not eating enough nutrients, or it could be because we need more nutrients than what would be considered standard to fight the inflammation in our bodies. I would hypothesize it's a little bit of both, given that 90 percent of Americans are deficient in certain vitamins and minerals, and on top of that our bodily needs are higher due to inflammatory stress.

If all of this feels like a bit too much information, just remember this: Endo is not is a single-faceted issue, is not a simple gynecological problem, and is not confined to your pelvic cavity. These points are incredibly important to understand as we discuss holistic healing because diet and lifestyle changes are critical when addressing immune system regulation, reverse malnutrition, healing and sealing the gut, and hormone balance.

Miriam's Story

I was 19 when I first went to the hospital with excruciating pain in my pelvis. They asked me to pee in a cup, told me nothing was wrong, and sent me home. This was my first time in the hospital and, being so young, I went home embarrassed for causing a scene.

I spent the next 18 years attending yoga classes, visiting naturopaths, traditional Chinese medicine practitioners, doctors, gynecologists, healers, massage therapists, and more. Naturopaths gave me supplements I didn't feel I could absorb. Doctors prescribed me contraceptives or other drugs I wanted to avoid since, for me, they often came with nasty side effects. Eventually I stopped talking about it, which is easier when you don't know what "it" is, anyway.

I had an assortment of episodes over the years: collapsing in agonizing pain, fainting, vomiting, sweating profusely, and diarrhea. Every 15 days I was a different person; I felt angry, emotional, bloated, exhausted, and at times I just felt like smashing my head into a wall. During my period I would pump myself full of painkillers and get on with it.

At 37, after tearfully begging, my GP finally referred me to a new gynecologist (the previous one had told me my symptoms weren't connected). Within minutes she said, "I'm sure you're riddled with endometriosis. We'll go in and have look." She examined me and I received a diagnosis: stage IV. Severe. Finally, at the age of 38 and after nearly 20 years of pushing for an answer, I had one. It turns out that it wasn't all in my head.

THE MOST COMMON SYMPTOMS

The most common symptoms of endo usually involve cyclical pain, abnormal cycles, and infertility. Cyclical pain is pain at menstruation, ovulation, or both. The pain can be anywhere on the spectrum from very uncomfortable to severe. Many of us were told that period pain or cramps are normal, so it's important to note here that painful periods are common but are *not normal.* Many women with endo have abnormally heavy cycles, although they can also be abnormally light—both are important to note. And as far as fertility, between 30 and 50 percent of endometriosis patients will deal with infertility at some point, which I'll discuss further.

Beyond cyclical pain, there are other types of pelvic pain commonly associated with endometriosis: dyspareunia (painful sex) and pain with bowel movements or bladder emptying. This could be due directly to endometriosis growth on your organs, or as an associated effect of pelvic inflammation, gut inflammation, dysbiosis, or pelvic floor or core dysfunction.

Gastrointestinal symptoms are so common in our community that we have a word for it: endo-belly. This is the slang term for the enormous bloating or gastric distress that often accompanies endometriosis. Ninety-three percent of women with endo present with GI issues of some kind—anywhere from chronic bloating and indigestion to an inflammatory bowel syndrome diagnosis and serious pain associated with digestion. This makes sense considering that endometriosis is partially a gut-related issue.

OTHER SYMPTOMS

Body mechanics may also play a role with endo. Many women with endometriosis have back pain, hip pain, or even knee or ankle pain, as well as a misplaced (retroverted, tipped, or retroflexed) uterus. They often have pelvic floor or core dysfunction, meaning they're moving and holding tension in ways that hurt rather than heal. These symptoms aren't necessarily caused by endo, but they can directly contribute to more pain through restricted blood flow and abnormal pressure in the pelvic cavity.

Other associated symptoms include chronic fatigue, brain fog, depression, and anxiety. Chronic fatigue was one of my personal battles with this disease, and I don't know how many times I Googled "why so tired endometriosis."

Because we're all unique, and endometriosis can manifest in so many ways, you may notice that your symptoms rarely line up exactly with those of other endo patients. Consequently, your own path to healing will be just as unique as your disease, so never judge your healing journey by another's.

THE ENDO–INFERTILITY CONNECTION

Endometriosis is connected to fertility blues for a variety of reasons, and it's estimated that 30 to 50 percent of women with endo will suffer from infertility at some point.

Some women may be able to conceive but suffer from recurrent miscarriages due to the inflammatory nature of the pelvis, adhesions, scarring, or other endo-related issues. Other women with endo may require medical assistance to help them conceive and carry a pregnancy to term. Endometriosis in its advanced stages may cause irreversible damage to the ovaries or fallopian tubes, physically inhibiting the ability to conceive naturally without assisted reproductive technology. Early diagnosis is key with endo and fertility.

There is another, more confusing side of infertility for endo-women, and that's unexplained infertility: You haven't gotten pregnant in more than a year, and there's no reason you shouldn't be pregnant. You are ovulating and menstruating, you have clear fallopian tubes, and all your mechanics are a go. Yet nothing is happening.

Some of the biggest pregnancy inhibitors accounting for unexplained infertility include malnutrition, blood sugar dysregulation, chronic stress, gut infections, hormonal imbalances, thyroid issues, and lack of blood flow to the pelvis. These issues can be addressed by the holistic diet and lifestyle approach presented in this book.

Two of the biggest pregnancy inhibitors—chronic stress and blood sugar dysregu-lation—both have a similar effect on the body: They raise cortisol, a steroid hormone that regulates a wide range of processes, including immune response and blood sugar regulation. Because your adrenal glands are responsible for making both cortisol and sex hormones, they will always (smartly) prioritize cortisol over reproduction in case you're in a fight-or-flight moment—like running from an escaped lion at the zoo. Reducing starches and sugars in your diet while increasing protein and fat helps you balance your blood sugar, which then allows your overworked adrenals to sigh with relief. By simultaneously working on your mindfulness, reducing everyday stressors, and sleeping better, you'll have your adrenals feeling like they're on vacation. And you know what happens on vacation . . . wink, wink.

But balancing blood sugar is not a magic bullet for every endo sufferer. Recall that up to 93 percent of all endometriosis patients have deep-seated gut issues that may be limiting nutrient absorption and, when combined with the nutrient-poor diets so common in our society, they may end up deeply malnourished. In fact, the very nutrients women with endo have been shown to be deficient in are *vital* fertility nutrients, including vitamins E, C, D, and A, zinc, omega-3s, and selenium! Therefore, it's important to focus on gut health and a diet founded on a variety of nutrient-dense foods to reverse nutritional deficiencies.

Lastly, women do not shoulder all of the causes of infertility—let's not forget the sperm! Current research shows men's healthy sperm count has dropped a shocking 50 percent over the past 40 years. It takes two to tango, endometriosis or not.

Claire's Story

I was diagnosed with severe endometriosis and adenomyosis at 26. After puberty I suffered with a range of increasingly debilitating symptoms, such as severe period pain, bloating, and fatigue. When I finally had a laparoscopy in 2016 it was a relief to discover the cause of my suffering. I'd honestly thought I was dying, which wreaks havoc on your mental health and productivity!

I'd hoped to feel better after having my endometriosis excised, but although I had some reduction in my symptoms, I was still experiencing some discomfort and fatigue. I had also been trying for a baby for more than two years with no success.

During this time at rock bottom, I met Katie and began working on my diet to improve my symptoms. It was clear I needed to work on leveling out my blood sugar and on increasing my intake of healthy fats and minerals. Perhaps it was focusing on an abundance of goodness rather than deprivation, but I was amazed how easy it was and how quickly I started to feel truly well. For the first time in a decade I had the energy I needed to thrive. And most miraculous of all, exactly three months after starting my dietary changes I became pregnant naturally. I never thought this would be possible. Baby Barney is here now, and he reminds me every day of how precious health is, and how small, positive changes can change your life so much.

TREATMENTS

Because every endo-woman is unique, there's no one-size-fits-all approach to treatment. Sorting through the treatment options can often feel like a minefield because it entails weighing opinions from doctors, nutritionists, health coaches, surgeons, and endo community members.

The best approach for you will be the perfect mix of treatments based on your own disease and symptoms, and it may be a mix of medical, surgical, nutritional, and lifestyle changes. Resilience is key when a new approach doesn't yield the results you hoped for. Keep seeking the treatment option that works for you!

Here's an overview of treatments.

CONVENTIONAL MEDICAL APPROACHES

Medical treatments to manage endometriosis symptoms include hormone therapy and painkillers as needed. Hormonal therapies include oral contraceptives, the Mirena coil, Lupron, or gonadotropin-releasing hormone (GnRH) analogues. All these options can minimize symptoms, but none actually treat endo. Nor do they come without side effects. For some women, these side effects are unnoticeable compared to their symptom relief; for others, the side effects are so unbearable that they must seek other options.

Pain medication itself is a tricky field to navigate for the chronic pain community, since the side effects of certain medications may outweigh the benefits in the long run. Opioids, for example, are a dangerous class of painkillers to dabble with if you have chronic pain; the addiction rates (and associated deaths) are astounding. The better choices are NSAIDs (such as aspirin and ibuprofen) or acetaminophen, although continual use may damage the liver or degrade the stomach and/or intestinal lining over time, leading to ulcers, digestive insufficiency, and dysbiosis, and thereby furthering malnutrition and inflammatory stress. This is not about med-shaming; it's about informed consent (what I like to call med-ucation) so that patients can best understand the precautions they should take when regularly using pharmaceuticals.

SURGERY

To address the endometriosis itself, it's widely agreed that the best way remove lesions and restore organ integrity is through laparoscopic excision surgery (LAPEX) done by a specialist. This type of surgery is performed with a laser rather than the commonly used *ablation* technique that superficially burns the endometriosis lesions, potentially leaving remains that grow back. LAPEX has a high success rate for both reducing pain and limiting recurrence, and it is considered the gold standard within the medical community.

The problem that arises for the average sufferer is that there are relatively few endometriosis surgical specialists in the world, and LAPEX surgeries can be expensive. Thus, it will be up to you to weigh the costs and benefits of your own disease and symptom severity when considering surgery, and remember that although diet and lifestyle changes are a great help, there is sadly no stand-in for a surgery when you really need one.

ALTERNATIVE THERAPIES

Many women also find alternative and complementary therapies useful, including acupuncture, traditional Chinese medicine, yoga, meditation, physical therapy, and pelvic floor therapy. These therapies, which I discuss in greater depth in chapter 3, can help the endo-woman bring her body back to a place of balance. If you've tried one therapy and it didn't help much, try another.

FUNCTIONAL MEDICINE

One avenue of treatment I recommend considering for every endo sufferer is working with a functional medicine practitioner. These are clinically trained MDs who have received functional medicine training to seek out and treat the root cause of issues, rather than treating the symptoms. A perfect example might be an irritable bowel syndrome (IBS) diagnosis. Instead of prescribing laxatives or fiber, a functional medicine doctor might run a variety of stool and gut health tests to understand the root cause of why your digestive system isn't working properly, and then work with you to treat that issue so you can resolve your IBS symptoms rather than mask them. Few of us realize there are doctors like these out there who can help us heal. To find someone near you, check out paleophysiciansnetwork.com or ifm.org/find-a-practitioner/.

DIET AND LIFESTYLE

After successfully reversing my own debilitating endometriosis through diet and lifestyle changes, I've dedicated my life to helping other women in similar situations. There is no drug that balances hormones, regulates the immune system, heals and seals the gut lining, replenishes the fuel needed for an anti-inflammatory army, restores the uterus to the correct position, reverses malnutrition, removes endocrine-disrupting chemicals from your daily life, or allows you to genuinely smile. No, these are all achieved through targeted diet and lifestyle approaches. It's a system I've seen women use to reclaim their lives.

You still may need surgery, medical intervention, therapy, or more—endo is a complex disease that requires many types of care. Remember, healing from endo requires an approach that is holistic—one that uses all the tools in your toolkit to bring your body back into balance and that may require a mix of healing modalities. The journey is yours and there's empowerment in choosing your own path back to health.

Donna-Marie's Story

I battled with stage IV pelvic and rare umbilical endometriosis for several years. My main symptoms consisted of chronic pelvic pain, deep fatigue, and serious digestive disorders. I simply couldn't function day to day—I was a hopeless hormonal mess. In January 2017, I was on a mission to #EndEndo and I thank God that I happened on the Heal Endo diet and lifestyle approach. I finally felt empowered to make some serious healing shifts by focusing on lifestyle changes and good whole foods–based nutrition—much of which was contrary to the dietary advice that was circulating in the endo community.

It was a little scary to go against the grain (quite literally), but the evidence of others who had tried this approach was enough to drive me to give it a try with zero regrets. I have since discovered firsthand that food *is* medicine! Katie taught me how to use properly prepared, nutritious whole foods to calm and restore my extremely sick body. I removed my bloat, healed my digestive tract, leveled out my off-the-chart blood sugar levels, balanced my hormones, and reenergized my then very slow, toxic, depleted body with food. It's been truly amazing!

I no longer suffer from chronic pelvic pain or endo-belly, and my monthly cycles are lighter, shorter, and virtually pain-free. To complete my healing process, I combined my highly successful holistic efforts with a surgical procedure to remove the stubborn umbilical nodule, and now my future is truly healthy and bright.

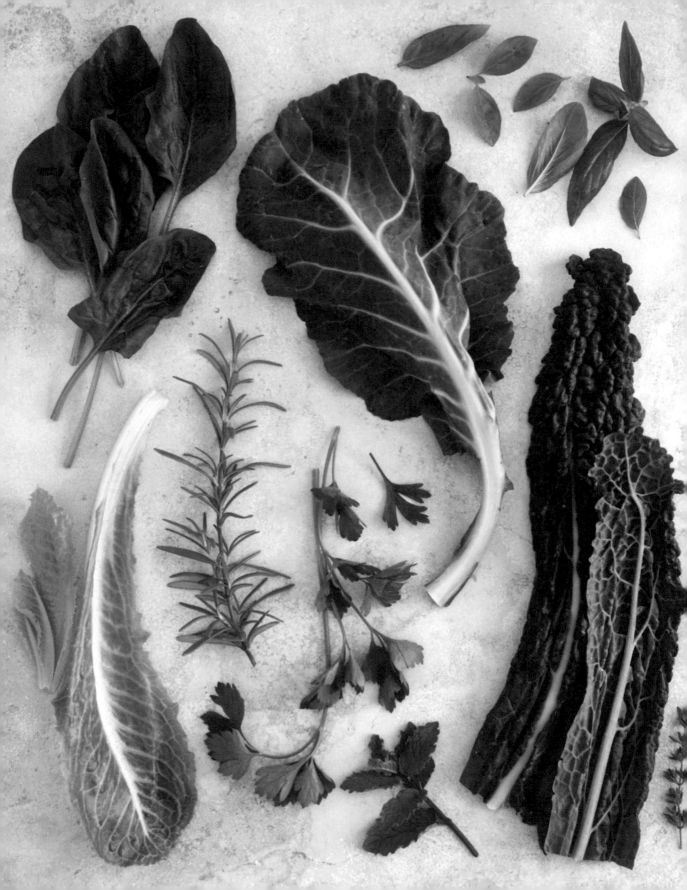

CHAPTER 2

Endometriosis and Nutrition

When I started dabbling with healing foods, I followed the traditional, extremely restrictive "endo diet" that most of us know, which seemingly hurt as much as it helped. In this diet, the main focus seemed to be restriction: no gluten, dairy, red meat, soy, caffeine, sugar, alcohol, or fun. Okay, I added the no fun, but that's what it felt like. Truth be told, a healing diet should fill you up, literally and figuratively. Yes, the triggers should be removed, but the focus should be nutrient infusion rather than a smorgasbord of gluten-free fare or "healthy" desserts. By focusing on refilling, we can support the body's ability to manage pain, inflammation, and other underlying health issues contributing to endo.

BLOOD SUGAR DYSREGULATION

It's probably 9 or 10 a.m., you're at work (or school), and you're huuuuungry. You have a few hours until lunch so you gobble a quick cereal bar. OMG, two hours later and you're starving again?! Lunch is so close, but so far—how about an apple? Lunch comes, you're not that hungry because you snacked, so you eat half your lunch—but now it's 2 p.m. and you're tired and hangry (hungry and angry), so you opt for a coffee . . . plus a little treat. At dinner and a small amount fills you up, so you definitely need a sweet treat from the freezer around 8 p.m.

Phew, another hungry day! This, ladies, is a textbook example of blood sugar dysregulation, and boy does it cause internal chaos.

Let's do a little exercise to better understand what blood sugar regulation really is: Imagine blood. See how sticky it is? That stickiness is sugar! Congratulations, you've met your blood sugar, and your body needs to keep that sugar at moderately low levels. Too much sugar and your blood turns to molasses; too little sugar and your cells starve. Which is exactly why this system keeps your blood sugar levels steady no matter what you eat. It's an incredible system.

Never have we had access to so many carbohydrates 24/7. In their simplest forms, all carbohydrates turn into sugar—glucose or fructose, scientifically. Although the excess sugars we most often think of are the processed refined varieties, they can also be what we think of as healthy foods: grains, bread, pasta, juices, beans, potatoes, and way too much fruit. If these carb-heavy (and therefore sugar-heavy) foods make up a small portion of your diet, no problem. However, if they're the *foundation* of your diet, they are causing your blood sugar to spike, leading to complications like systemic inflammation and stress on your hormonal system. Blood sugar dysregulation is the endo elephant in the room—it's something that contributes dramatically to endometriosis and inflammation symptoms, but in a society of sugar addicts, it's something too few of us are talking about.

Blood sugar dysregulation causes inflammation in an assortment of ways. Insulin is the helper hormone that delivers glucose (sugars) to cells. When there's too much glucose in the system, cells start to turn insulin away (called insulin resistance), but the insulin keeps beating on the proverbial cell door to get in. All that door-banging causes cellular inflammation, and when you're provoking a big insulin surge all day every day, it contributes to that body-wide inflammation you've been blaming on your pelvis. Also, excess sugars feed dysbiosis, something intricately connected to endometriosis. The more dysbiosis, the more inflammation, the bigger the endo-belly bloat, and the more endo lesions.

As for associated symptoms, the blood sugar roller coaster takes a toll on the endo-body. Chronic fatigue? High blood sugar drains your adrenals. Sluggish liver? The liver has no time to detoxify because it's stuck in the trenches balancing glucose levels. Unexplained infertility? Your body doesn't know if your stress is an advancing army or a blood sugar–spiking carrot juice, so to protect you from harm she promotes adrenaline instead of progesterone.

There's so much misinformation about endo and diets. I've seen many women accidentally make it worse by removing the very foods that balance blood sugar, namely protein and fat, and instead filling up on blood sugar–spiking fruits, starches, grains, or gluten-free choices instead. Many women I work with are easily eating 7 to

10 servings of fruit per day or filling up on "healthy" meals that more closely resemble dessert. They seem to be hungry 24/7. Insert painful endo-flair, drained energy, brain fog, chipped fingernails, brittle hair, and big endo-belly. Bummer.

This is why it's imperative to address this issue now. Lucky for us, balancing blood sugar is not rocket science. It's simply about filling up on tons of low-starch veggies, proteins, and fat first and foremost, while rounding out your meals with more limited amounts of fruit and starchy veggies. No, it doesn't mean you need to cut out all carbs. Yes, it does mean your taste buds and cooking habits will need to change. But if you approach these changes slowly and sustainably, you might be surprised just how fast you feel better.

I always recommend clients begin with breakfast. It's a meal that many women skip or for which they eat "breakfast dessert" and end up starving a few hours later—creating a rollercoaster of disaster for the rest of the day. The body can be vicious when holding onto its sweet addiction, so my hope is that you use the one-month meal plan as a guide to set you up for success, making incremental changes starting with your first meal of the day. You'll learn how easy (and delicious) it can be to live a sugar-balanced life.

GLUTEN AND DAIRY

Gluten and dairy are more widely recognized culprits in the endo community than blood sugar, but are still important to acknowledge. Many endo-women may still be eating these foods without realizing the direct effect on their endo.

Let's start with gluten, which I like to say is on the endo most-wanted list no matter who you are, your ancestry, or if you think you tolerate it just fine. If you have endo pain, endo-belly, or systemic inflammation, I don't believe you're tolerating gluten as fine as you think. In one study of women with endo, 75 percent of participants who cut out gluten had dramatic reductions in their pain from this change alone. This may be because gluten can poke holes in your intestinal lining as well as change your microbiome for the worse. Another study was able to illustrate how gluten increases inflammatory markers in *all* individuals, not just those with a diagnosed disease.

There are a host of reasons why someone with pain, inflammation, and gut issues would want to avoid dairy. It is, of course, quite allergenic, with between 1 and

4 percent of adults unable to tolerate any dairy at all, and between 25 and 75 percent of people are lactose-intolerant, depending on their ethnicity.

Beside allergies, dairy impacts the endo-body by affecting the gut and causing inflammation. Dairy products contain protease inhibitors, which may directly contribute to leaky gut and which can also hinder nutrient absorption—an important consideration when reversing malnutrition. They may also lend a hand in insulin resistance and thus inflammation (as you now know after learning about blood sugar). Plus, pasteurization itself can create an inflammatory response because of how it denatures proteins; these mutilated amino acids can create pro-inflammatory irritants that disturb the gut lining, which may be one reason more people are developing casein (milk protein) intolerance.

I must say that I'm a nutritional therapist who's not wholly against dairy, at least not when it comes from 100-percent grass-fed animals or A2 dairy products from certain cows or other dairy animals. Dairy from 100-percent grass-fed animals has CLA (conjugated linoleic acid, a type of anti-inflammatory fat), omega-3s, minerals, and fat-soluble vitamins, and might be a healthy option for some to include in their diet if (and only if) it's tolerated. Of course, if you suffer from endo and her associated symptoms at all, it's necessary to eliminate all dairy for at least one to three months or longer. You can then reintroduce some easier-to-digest options, like ghee and butter from grass-fed animals or goat or sheep cheese and yogurt, to see if you truly tolerate them.

For any naysayers out there who have tried eating gluten free or dairy free before and felt nothing improved (or you felt worse), this doesn't mean your body inherently loves gluten and dairy. This could be because: a) you didn't try it for a long enough period of time; b) you replaced gluten with a lot of gluten-free processed foods, which are still often gluten contaminated and don't offer your body the benefit it's after; or c) you have some significant dysbiosis going on, which may be why you felt worse replacing these foods with healthy options. Depending on the type of dysbiosis, you may react to many healthy foods, such as sweet potatoes, onions, garlic, and avocados, which is why some women "fall off the wagon" when approaching dietary changes because they felt better eating bread than veggies.

If dairy and gluten make up the bulk of your diet, this swap may seem overwhelming at first, especially when we realize they're hiding in many of our everyday packaged foods like soy sauce, marinades, condiments, and baked goods. Don't worry, eliminating them gets easier with time, especially as you learn to replace packaged foods overall with a diet focused on whole foods: veggies, fruits, animal proteins, and fat. This whole-foods diet is what will make you start to feel better, and feeling better is imperative if you're going to stick with these changes.

FATS

F-A-T, a three-letter word that provokes so many emotions. We need healthy fats for cognitive function, to calm inflammation, and for energy and stamina. Yet over the past decade information has become skewed on this topic and the truth has become cloudy. So let me set you up for cellular success with some endo fat-ucation.

Harmful fats will make your overall health, and endo, worse. They include the well-known enemy trans fats as well as vegetable oils such as canola (rapeseed), safflower, sunflower, grape-seed, corn, soy, margarine, and most vegan butters, many of which are pushed as "healthy" but are truly not due to the manufacturing process that renders them extremely toxic. These butters are made using high heat and a toxic gas called hexane to create rancid oil, which is made palatable with bleaching and deodorizing. Using these butters is akin to pouring damaging free radicals over your food, leading to endo-disaster.

Healing fats, on the other hand, are ancestral foods that deliver fat-soluble vitamins, create slow-burning energy for blood sugar regulation, support fertility, and offer the foundational building blocks for each cell in your body. They also make food taste delicious. They include butter, ghee, lard, tallow, extra-virgin olive oil, coconut oil, palm oil, and certain nut and seed oils. Food sources include egg yolks, coconut, fatty cuts of meat, nuts, seeds, avocados, coldwater fish, and roe. Saturated fats are the building blocks of all of your sex hormones, whereas omega-3 fats directly contribute to your body's anti-inflammatory response. If you don't have enough omega-3s in your diet, you won't have enough in your body. It's that simple.

To avoid harmful varieties of fat, learn to read labels and avoid any of the above list. Doing so will mean tossing most salad dressings, condiments, and packaged foods (which are usually stuffed to the brim with veggie oils), and replacing them with homemade items or brands like Paleo Leap that use ancestral fats in sauces and dressings. I also recommend buying good-quality oils, even if that means you can only afford one or two varieties at a time. Doing so will help your skin, your energy, your brain function, and your overall quality of life. This is why if you want to imagine rebuilding your body cell by cell, you must ensure you include all the ancestral fats you can tolerate. Never fear good fats.

Is Red Meat the Enemy?

The short answer is no. But factory-farmed red meat might be—even when it's organic. On the other hand, 100-percent grass-fed meats and organs are nutrient dense and full of anti-inflammatory omega-3s, CLA, glycine, and the most absorbable forms of zinc and iron—two minerals we're often deficient in. When animals are 100 percent grass-fed (the 100 percent is important when checking labels), they benefit the land, combat climate change (called regenerative agriculture), and reverse malnutrition. So, although I agree that factory-farmed meat should be avoided for health, animal welfare, and environment, remember that 100-percent grass-fed animals are totally different. Any time you see eggs or any kind of meat in a recipe in this book, I mean from 100-percent grass-fed animals.

FODMAPS, HISTAMINES, AND OTHER TRIGGERS

If you feel like you've tried every diet under the sun to no avail, read this section closely. There are real reasons why supposedly healthy foods could make you feel worse rather than better. Any or all of these culprits may be blocking your recovery more than you realize.

FODMAPS

FODMAPs in an acronym for fermentable carbohydrates called oligosaccharides, disaccharides, monosaccharides, and polyols. These are complex names for certain types of sugars in foods that feed bacteria, which is awesome if you have a normal, healthy gut microbiome. If you have bad bacterial overgrowth, though, those sugars may be feeding the wrong bacteria in the wrong places. When this happens, healthy foods like apples, onions, garlic, sweet potatoes, and others can bloat you like a balloon, cause chronic nausea, constipation, diarrhea, or both, and make your life generally miserable.

FODMAP intolerance is often linked to both IBS and endometriosis, perhaps because of their association to a form of dysbiosis called small-intestinal bacterial overgrowth (SIBO). SIBO is what happens when bacteria flourishes where it shouldn't, such as your small intestine, and wreaks havoc when you eat high-FODMAP foods. This leads to both chronic inflammation and leaky gut.

A study in the medical journal *JAMA* detected SIBO in up to 84 percent of IBS cases, and another small study in *Fertility and Sterility* found that 80 percent of women with endo who also presented with terrible gastrointestinal issues tested positive for SIBO. If you suspect this is you, consider following a strict low-FODMAP diet for two to four weeks and see if you notice improvements. If you do, work with a professional to get tested to see if you have a gut infection that can be treated once and for all.

HISTAMINE INTOLERANCE

We now know that endometriosis lesions contain more mast cells than normal cells do, and this has uncovered a new area of study for the endo sufferer. Mast cells produce histamines, those little buggers that cause you to itch, swell, and become inflamed. It's part of a normal immune response in healthy people, but if you're reacting unnecessarily to histamines they can cause systemic issues like allergies, migraines, digestive problems, rashes, asthma, or even continuously flare your endo.

Like FODMAP intolerance, histamine intolerance may also be linked to dysbiosis. A healthy person should break down histamines in the gut with a specific enzyme called diamine oxidase (DAO). In certain people, DAO can be severely lacking; they can simultaneously have an overgrowth of histamine-producing bacteria, and thus they can have excessive histamines flooding their body provoking that systemic inflammatory response. If you suspect this is you, following a low-FODMAP diet for two to four weeks may determine if histamines are a trigger, since research shows a low-FODMAP diet may reduce histamines by eightfold. If you need extra support, a strict low-histamine diet may be worth considering for a short period, or working with a professional who can help you uncover the underlying causes of these issues.

OTHER TRIGGERS

If you have a case of increased intestinal permeability (or leaky gut), you may be reacting to a slew of healthy foods you eat every day as they cross the gut barrier and end up directly in your bloodstream. This prompts your immune system to mount an attack against this food—something that should never happen—and is one reason the immune system becomes dysregulated in the first place. This may also be why you've become perplexed at how many foods you react to daily, even in mysterious ways like autoimmune flaring, joint pain, inflammation, insomnia, depression, and chronic fatigue. Reactionary foods here may include grains, beans, eggs, dairy, soy, alcohol, nuts, seeds, and nightshades (tomatoes, white potatoes, peppers, eggplant, etc.), items that may make up the bulk of your diet currently, and that must be removed short term in order to truly heal and seal your gut. Examples of this style of gut-healing diet include Gut and Psychology Syndrome (GAPS), Wahls, and the Paleo Autoimmune Protocol (AIP)—all strict elimination diets lasting one to three months.

HOW TO APPROACH

Although there is some overlap between these elimination diets, they're all quite unique in the issues they address, and therefore what foods they eliminate. This is why you may have tried one diet and felt no relief, or even felt worse. It's also why diets can seem so confusing when you're doing your best to eat well. You may be reacting to foods in all three categories, making you sometimes feel like you're losing your mind (believe me, you're not). What these diets do have in common is that they're meant to be short-term therapeutic diets, with the goal of reintroduction. So again, if you feel better using these diets as a guide but can't seem to rebound after, I recommend finding a specialist to work with to really address your unique set of symptoms.

If you feel you relate to a FODMAP or histamine intolerance, consider using the included recipes in this book as an aid for a two- to four-week elimination diet to see if that improves symptoms. Look for the low FODMAP (or substitutions) symbol as a guide. And if you're interested in learning more about endometriosis, dysbiosis, and leaky gut, check out the Resources section (see page 156).

HEALING FOODS

There is no endo diet that works for everyone, but there is a foundational framework we can all follow: vegetable-based, rich in omega-3s, low to moderate carbohydrates, as organic and local as possible, and with a focus on nutrient diversity and anti-inflammatory phytonutrients. This is similar to a Paleo diet, or a modified Mediterranean diet, minus the grains, where your focus is tons of fresh veggies (seven to nine cups per day), wild-caught coldwater fish, 100-percent grass-fed or pastured animals (snout to tail, meaning all parts of the animal rather than just ground meat or chicken breast), fresh herbs, plus ancestral fats and a bit of fruit for fun.

This emphasis on veggies and herbs is important for numerous reasons. First of all, they are full of antioxidant-rich vitamins, minerals, and the array of phytonutrients known for their anti-inflammatory and gut-healing properties. Studies show that a diet rich in phytonutrients can help reduce or even reverse gut dysbiosis, and lucky for us we can increase our consumption of these compounds right now by consuming an abundance of fresh veggies, fruits, herbs, and certain teas.

The other healing aspect of a veggie-based diet is the amount of fiber it contains to feed your gut microbiome. Sadly, most of us are fiber-deficient, eating about half our quota and with much of that fiber coming from starchy and nutrient-poor grain-based foods. The better way to increase fiber, vitamins, minerals, and antioxidants is to instead focus on the rainbow of veggies, and your gut microbiome will thank you.

This diet also emphasizes eating to reverse malnutrition and substantially increasing your omega-3 fat consumption. Instead of replacing your packaged favorites with "organic, gluten-free" processed alternatives, you actually replace them with nutrient-dense bombs. This includes seafood like fatty coldwater fish, shellfish, 100-percent grass-fed meats, organ meats, and rich bone broths, plus every color of plant under the sun.

Many of these foods in substance or quantity may sound confusing, foreign, or downright scary to you right now. Please don't panic. This is why you have this book to guide you! I've helped many women switch their diet foundations (and yes, their taste buds too) over the years, and I have faith that with the right attitude and excitement, you can too. Remember, it's about sustainable change, so be patient and have fun on the journey.

Erin's Story

During my worst struggles with endo, I had big plans for the future that I fully believed would never come to pass. I was comatose with chronic fatigue, and had been for so long that I couldn't imagine life any other way. To start addressing this unimaginable weight of symptoms, I started small, by adding bone broth and sauerkraut into my diet for nutrients and gut health. I started walking 10 minutes a day. Soon after, we added more—a trip to the farmer's market for veggies, a 15-minute walk, and cutting out dairy. Every couple of weeks I made tiny shifts; either increasing my walks, adding nutrient-dense liver and fish eggs to my ever-changing diet, or finding energy to cook more meals. My body was starved for nutrients, so we focused on loading it with grass-fed meats, vegetables, targeted supplements, and herbal teas. I began seeing a pelvic floor physical therapist and increased my walking time.

Two months into our program, I noticed my chronic fatigue starting to lift. I walked and cooked more. Five months after that, I went to Israel—a dream trip of mine. I did everything I wanted to without collapsing from fatigue! Now I'm in nursing school and amazed I can keep up with the grueling schedule and long days on campus and at the hospital. All of this I credit to the Heal Endo diet and lifestyle approach—a lifestyle that gave me my life back! A year ago I never would have believed myself capable of all the things I am doing now. It's truly a miracle.

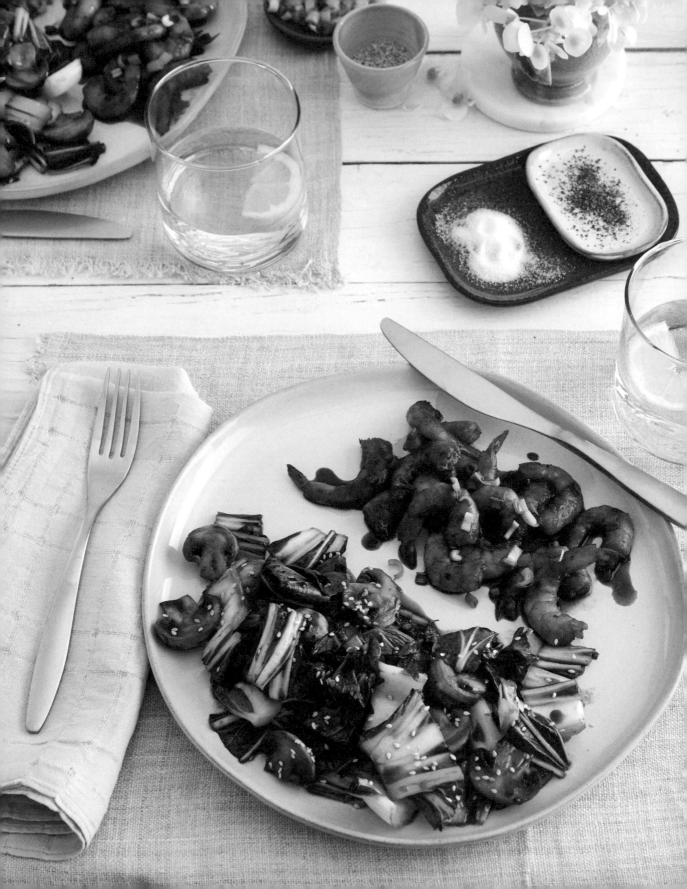

CHAPTER 3

Endometriosis and Lifestyle

As a nutritional therapist I wish I could say diet is everything when it comes to healing, but it's not. Diet can't address the deep-seated stress of your life, the lack of movement or body misalignment, the missing sleep, the lack of social ties, or the time spent on screens. These all add up to create pain and tension in the endo-body, and must be addressed to truly build better health. Fortunately, by working to minimize these excess body stressors, you'll find yourself living a life you're much happier with! And happiness is everything when it comes to holistic healing.

MEAL SPACING

Meal spacing is perhaps one of the most important endo lifestyle factors you've never heard of. Simply, it means eating full and balanced meals, three to four times per day, with no snacking in between. No sipping coffee and cream or green juices, no nibbling on nuts or crackers to tide you over, just simply drinking filtered water and calmly waiting for your next meal in four to five hours. Did you just faint? Maybe. If you deal with blood sugar regulation issues or have strong mental ties to snacking, this may seem like an unreachable goal.

Why meal space? Because it's imperative to your digestion, your hormones, and your success in implementing this new whole-foods diet. Our bodies didn't evolve to eat all the time, and your digestive system needs a break. Moreover, it's only when your digestive system isn't working that your liver can focus on other issues, like detoxifying. So, if you're munching all day long you'll run out of digestive mojo, and your body rarely has time to clean up shop.

Meal spacing helps balances the hormones ghrelin and leptin, your "hungry" and "full" hormones, and if you're never listening to them you're actually contributing to the hormonal chaos. Plus, allowing yourself to get really good and hungry (not hangry) will push your taste buds to be more open to new foods. If you snack your hunger into submission with hyper-palatable snacks, your body may just never be hungry enough for whole-foods meals.

Meal spacing won't happen overnight, though. Go as slow as you need to, knowing that the more you eat at meals, the longer you'll go to your next. Make it a one- to three-month goal, starting with a solid breakfast so that you can complete your meal-spacing marathon all the way to lunch.

STRESS RELIEF

Stress is linked not only to increased gut permeability, mental health issues, and disease prevalence, but also to the severity of endometriosis. Researchers analyzed rats with endo by putting them through a stressful swim test for 10 days to measure the effects. This high-stress activity not only increased the amount of inflammation involved with the endo *and* surrounding tissues, it also increased the number of endometriosis lesions! We might as well call it "stress-o-metriosis," since chronic, debilitating stress isn't just common, it's the new norm.

The problem with chronic stress is that our bodies haven't evolved to handle it. They evolved to handle a specific stress—being chased by a lion, facing famine one winter—but not unrelenting disaster news, the workplace, body image pressure, the exorbitant cost of living, or even just that nasty commute. So when we face these stressors every day without knowing how to turn them off, we start to live in a state of chronic stress. Our faces screw up, our shoulders hunch, our bellies tighten, our breath is shallow, and . . . our endo flares.

This is why addressing this issue head-on will help you shed your worries and, at the same time, shed some of that endo pain. It's a win-win! Some ways to help are actually pretty simple, and you can begin right now. Meditation, deep breathing, and guided imagery are all awesome ways to start, as they help pull your head back into the "now," rather than grinding away about what your boss said yesterday. Plus, there are great apps to help you take the guesswork out of these modalities, such as the Calm app, meditations, music, and even sleep stories to help you start calming down.

SLEEP

Increasing sleep quality and quantity is the easiest thing you can do today. The problem is that most of us don't prioritize this restorative healing time. In fact, the average amount of sleep Americans get has declined two hours per night since the 1960s and that 730 fewer hours (90 full nights) of sleep per year has been linked to a rise in chronic disease. Sleep is the time your body detoxifies, repairs, and cleans house, so if your night janitors are taking three months off, you're kind of screwed.

Luckily, reprioritizing sleep isn't hard for most of us when the main culprit is a screen, whether its Netflix, social media, or work. Removing all screens two hours before bed and doing something restorative instead is a much better solution. Pick up the lost art of reading a book, the hobby you used to enjoy, or chatting with your partner. If you truly need to be on screens, blue light–blocking glasses (they're cheap on Amazon) can really help remove some of the light stimulation and help you fall asleep faster.

For some of us with endo, the associated symptoms of anxiety, depression, stress, or pain-somnia can keep us awake. In these cases, make sleep your priority before *anything* else in this book. Focus on mindfulness, slowing way down, and perhaps even working with a professional, because you can't accomplish much of anything (healing least of all) if you're chronically sleep deprived.

MOVEMENT

Movement and alignment are key tenets of my Heal Endo message, and are quite different than exercise. Movement is the opposite of sedentariness, and alignment is a body moving correctly. When your body is sedentary or out of alignment, it may be weak or in pain, but it also means circulation is decreased. Without proper circulation to your pelvis, glutes, and core—the muscles usually atrophied from a lifestyle of sitting too much—you won't allow nutrients, immune activity, or hormones to reach their prime destination: your pelvic cavity. This directly affects endo, since research shows menstrual cramps are much worse when blood flow is restricted in the pelvic cavity.

Additionally, many if not all of us with endo have core or pelvic floor dysfunction of some sort. This means we're not moving properly or, even worse, moving in ways that hurt rather than help and may be why you have a misplaced uterus (tipped, retroverted, or otherwise). This is why I recommend moving more and moving better before doing anything else to support your healing anew.

The most affordable way to start is simply to walk more overall, and more frequently throughout the day. If you sit often, set a timer to walk five minutes every half hour to keep that blood flowing to your pelvis. Walk outside for nature bonus points. Also, consider getting a referral to a pelvic floor physical therapist or core recovery specialist who can help you retrain your musculature, breathe, and release tension. Relearning to move correctly may benefit your life—and pain—more than you ever could have imagined.

Don't Make It Worse

Please be careful when considering which movement is best for you! Remember that movement is supposed to help you feel better rather than create further problems. Always listen to your body and, when in doubt, talk to your doctor.

If addressing alignment or core dysfunction sounds nebulous, there are some really cool programs to help you get there—and you can do them from the comfort of your own home.

MoveU: This is one my favorite endo recommendations to retrain your body to breathe, move, and use your core correctly, all from the comfort of your own home. The group teaching this course excels at helping people with every type of alignment and/or pain issue get back on track through fun, yet comprehensive online videos, workouts, personal video analysis, and more. www.moveu.com

Restore Your Core: This 13-week program helps you learn how to move correctly and retrain your core musculature. It's designed by women for women with pelvic floor, core, and alignment issues, and therefore women with endometriosis. www.laurenohayon.com/offerings/restore-your-core/

Nutritious Movement: If you want some quick alignment and movement ideas, this is the place for bite-size info and videos. This innovative approach combines biomechanics, alignment, and natural movement, and is amazingly effective at helping you move better, and happier, once and for all. www.nutritiousmovement.com

SUPPLEMENTS AND ALTERNATIVE THERAPIES

There is an awesome assortment of alternative therapies to help women with endo through stress reduction, detoxification, and supporting healing pathways. Here are some of them.

TRADITIONAL CHINESE MEDICINE (TCM)

These ancient healing techniques include acupuncture, massage, and herbs, and may be a helpful non-invasive option for pain, infertility, blood flow, stress, and other endo-related symptoms. TCM conceptualizes endometriosis as a "blood stasis" condition, meaning circulation is poor (sound familiar?), and aims to support healing by lowering stress, increasing blood flow, and balancing hormones. Research published in 2018 in the *Chinese Journal of Integrative Medicine* has shown that TCM "can inhibit the postoperative recurrence of EM, improve quality of life, shorten the time to conception and increase pregnancy rates."

MAGNESIUM

Ideally, we should get our minerals from food. But magnesium is one mineral that seems to be in low supply. That's because our soils are quite depleted, and so too is our food. Combined with the fact that bodies under stress deplete magnesium like wildfire, many women with endo can be extremely in need. Deficiency can even exacerbate pain, since magnesium helps with muscle soothing and relaxation. If you and your doctor decide supplementation is appropriate, some of the most absorbable forms are magnesium glycinate or magnesium orotate. Although magnesium citrate (more commonly found) is less absorbable, it may still be an aid for the endo-woman in helping with regular or less-painful bowel movements.

DETOXIFICATION SUPPORT

We should be happily taking out cellular waste every day (also known as detoxing). But when our bodies become overburdened, over-toxic, or over-estrogenic, we often need extra support. To take the burden off your liver, consider supportive modalities like dry skin brushing (you literally brush your dry skin with a scrub-style brush to increase circulation and lymph flow to the surface of the skin), warm Epsom salt baths, oral oil pulling (an Ayurvedic detoxing practice where you swish sesame or coconut oil in your mouth for 10 to 20 minutes to draw out toxins), increased daily movement, or a good old-fashioned sweat (followed by a shower).

ARVIGO MAYA ABDOMINAL MASSAGE

This massage technique may help loosen or minimize scar tissue, adhesions, or cysts. It may even be able to place a tipped or retroverted uterus into the correct position while increasing proper blood flow to the abdominal cavity. This would provide increased circulation to bring in nutrients to support healthy tissues and hormonal function. Learn more at arvigotherapy.com.

Angie's Story

Before I began addressing my endo my typical day started at 4 a.m. after five or six hours of sleep. I would quickly eat breakfast and experience bloating and stomach upset. I was tired all day and brain fog was normal for me. I had been dealing with endometriosis and gut issues for years, and recently had suffered two miscarriages, which brought on a huge fear of trying to get pregnant again.

Desperate to heal, I finally decided I needed to make some huge changes, and immediately began to work on my diet, stress levels, sleep, and exercise. Due to the overly restricted diet I had myself on previously, I began to focus more on variety, including more vegetables than I had ever imagined. I was eating greens and squash for breakfast!

For lifestyle, I slowly worked up to seven to eight hours of sleep each night. Because I'm a personal trainer, I'd used exercise to cope with stress for years, without realizing it was stressing me out and exhausting me more than helping. My new focus was on recovery and taking my body out of the red zone I had planted it in. My stomach immediately started to relax.

My husband and toddler jumped on board as well. The diet was good for all of us and we had fun doing kitchen "experiments" trying new veggies. All of this was a critical part of my healing, plus having my family on board to embrace our new road to health. Today I feel like I reclaimed my life and my health through diet and lifestyle alone. A year ago I didn't even know that was possible.

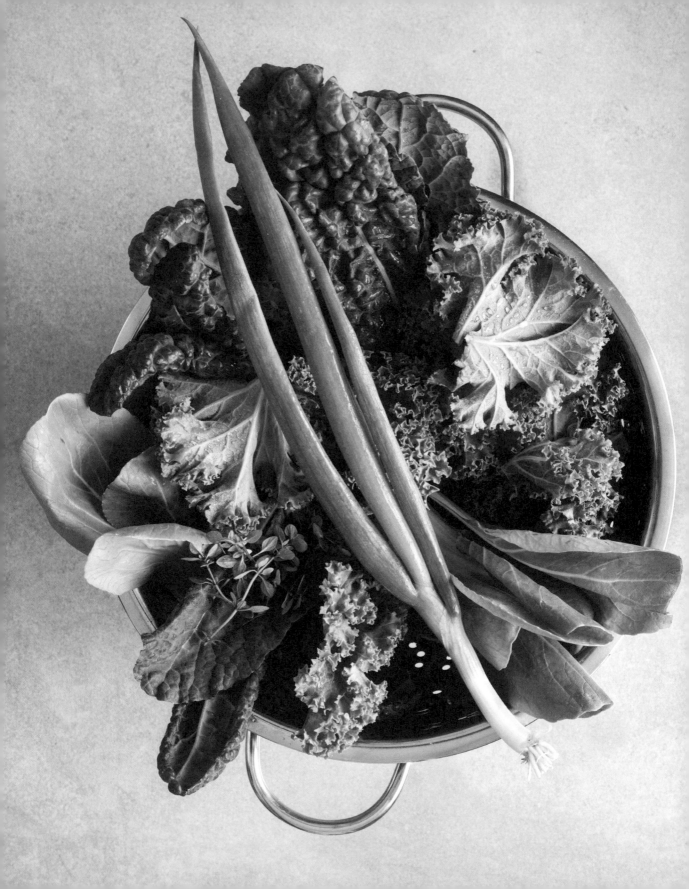

The Diet Plan

As you learned in part I, every endo sufferer will have a unique presentation of symptoms, which is exactly why there's no one specific endo diet for everyone. Nevertheless, there are important dietary strategies everyone can benefit from. I'll list them here in part II, along with an easy-to-use four-week plan to get you eating a nutrient-dense, whole-foods diet in one month. This diet framework is delicious, and is designed to reverse malnutrition, balance blood sugar, and get you to fewer days of discomfort every month.

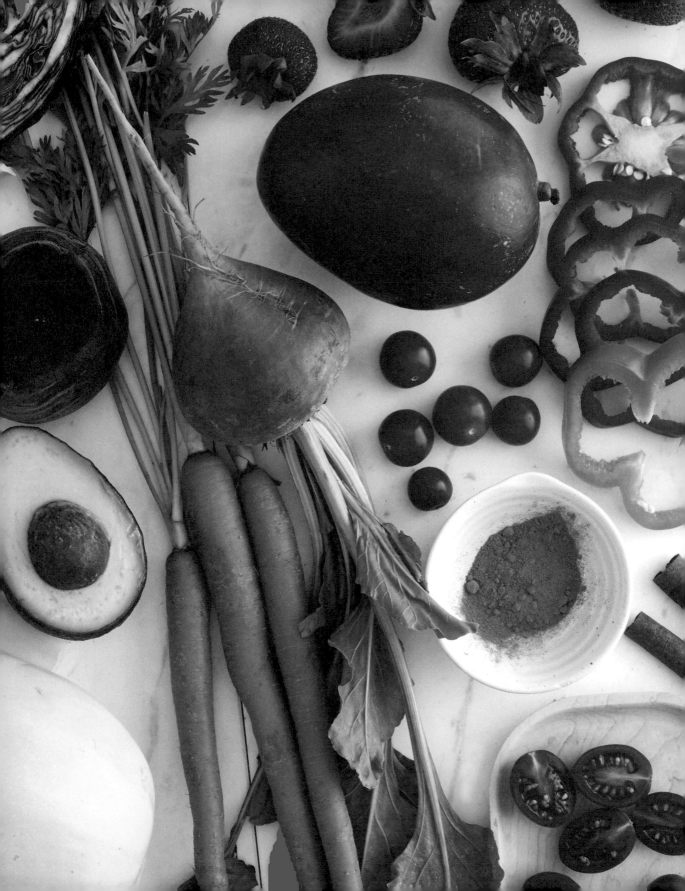

CHAPTER 4

Understanding the Endometriosis Diet

The diet presented in this book is built on the foods you need to rebuild a healthy body. It's a vegetable-based, omega-3, and antioxidant-rich dietary program based on whole foods, with an emphasis on abundance rather than restriction. Because this is a new paradigm of cooking for many people who rely on grains or processed foods to fill out their meals, the diet plan here is designed to help you make sustainable changes, starting with breakfast, your strategic blood sugar ally. Every week we'll add more whole foods to your diet—including using batch cooking to save time—until you suddenly have mastered three meals per day and are meeting or exceeding your recommended daily allowance (RDA) of essential nutrients every day. Ready? Set? Go!

THE DIET PLAN

The goal of this plan is to help you understand exactly what a diet so rich in veggies; wild, pastured, or grass-fed meats; and healthy fats looks like, and how you can achieve this in your own life. I want you to feel confident in the kitchen, following your taste buds rather than calories, and conquering batch cooking once and for all. I want you to be able to pinpoint which foods make you feel well and which ones may not. And I want you to break up with your addiction to sweet tastes once and for all with a gradual refocus on low-starch veggies.

Although I am against restriction in its traditional sense (calories, fat, flavor), this diet plan does eliminate common triggers such as gluten, soy, vegetable oils, sugar, peanuts, and processed dairy. Additionally, there won't be "gray area" foods such as beans, grains, or grass-fed dairy. These foods may not be inherently bad if you truly tolerate them and eat them in moderation, rather than using them to replace your nutrient-dense alternatives, but I leave that for you to decide. And although eggs are a gray area food as well (you truly may react), I keep them in a few breakfast recipes because they are so incredibly nutrient dense. Always remember to be cautious and listen to your body.

As you look over the meals included in this next month's meal plans, I'd like to emphasize that the recipes chosen are particularly helpful for addressing endometriosis symptoms. They utilize foods containing the most anti-inflammatory and immune-supporting nutrients per calorie we endo-gals so dearly need—omega-3s, phytonutrients, vitamins A and D—and it's why I suggest that, even if some of the ingredients are new or nerve-wracking (like liver or sardines), you give them a try! Of course, if you're nervous or just plain grossed out, you are welcome to substitute any recipe or ingredient for others in the book. I'm a firm believer that lifestyle changes should be done as slowly as needed in order to commit your body to the process.

This book's recipes swap some common staples for less common ones and swap processed foods for whole foods. The focus is on the process of making home-cooked meals with lots of flavor and without a lot of fancy. You can add fancy in at any time, but first things first: basic, healthy, tasty foods. They will begin to refuel your body without pushing your time or energy constraints to their limits.

To achieve these goals, the diet plan in the book will build on itself, starting with breakfast. In Week One, we will plan and prep seven days of breakfasts that are blood sugar–friendly and very nutrient dense (fiber, vitamins, minerals, antioxidants, fats, proteins, boom!). Focus here first, with the goal to eat as much as necessary to make it at least three hours (although four to five hours is ideal) until your next meal or snack, and then carry on with your day as usual.

Week Two and Week Three will add more whole foods in the form of some dinners and lunches. You will focus on a few rounds of batch cooking to see just how amazingly simple it is to prepare whole foods and have them available in your refrigerator so you never feel hungry or as if you just *have* to reach for chips. These weeks you may still decide to incorporate some old familiar foods, but the goal is to slowly step away from processed or sweet fillers as your taste buds and gut microbiome shift back to center, and you find yourself with fewer cravings.

Week Four will put it all together—three filling meals per day for meal spacing (consider four if you need it), and an example of a week of eating that is the definition of everything I preach: nutrient dense, veggie based, sugar balanced, and, most importantly, delicious.

As a general rule, if you know you react to any foods listed in this book, please don't use them just because I say they're "healthy." Also, if you want to use this book as an outline for a low-FODMAP diet, look for the substitutions or omissions under each recipe and adjust accordingly.

At the end of this month I hope you not only find yourself a more confident cook, but also find you have more energy, more stamina, less pain, and increased hope. Although holistic changes add up over time, you may feel a whole lot better even with just basic increases in your healthful food intake.

PREPARING YOUR KITCHEN

Preparation is the key to success in all aspects of whole-foods cooking. To avoid succumbing to the temptation of packaged snacks, you need to have the essentials in your pantry for tasty cooking, and extra food or snacks in the refrigerator and freezer to reheat in a jiffy. If you're chronically ill (or short on time), having the right tools will also be essential. As they say, time is money, and simple kitchen investments may be your sink or swim when switching your diet foundations. Affordability tip: Check garage sales, thrift shops, or Craigslist for kitchen items, or even ask family members who may be desperate to give certain items away.

STOCK YOUR PANTRY

Processed foods are often hyper-flavored, and why you may think whole foods are boring. Au contraire. I would argue it's your pantry that's boring, because quality ingredients and spices are truly the flavor of life. You don't have to buy all of these at once, but over the course of the month, work to stock your pantry with your favorite flavor-makers to set your meals up for success:

- **Fats:** coconut oil, extra-virgin olive oil, sesame oil, pastured lard or tallow, and 100-percent grass-fed ghee or butter, if you tolerate them

- **Herbs and spices:** Unrefined sea or Himalayan salt (please throw away *all* refined or iodized salt), black pepper, garlic powder, fresh ginger, onion powder, cinnamon, paprika, mint, thyme, basil, Italian seasoning, red pepper flakes, lemongrass, kaffir lime leaf, and cayenne pepper

- **For baking:** almond flour, coconut flour, raw honey, pure maple syrup, raw cacao powder, dark chocolate chips, coconut cream

- **Nuts:** raw almonds, cashews, macadamias, walnuts, pistachios, Brazil nuts, and/or pine nuts

- **Essentials:** coconut aminos (this will replace soy sauce), tomato paste and crushed tomatoes (preferably in glass jars), simple coconut milk (meaning without guar gum or other fillers), salsa, olives, balsamic vinegar, Dijon mustard, apple cider vinegar, rice vinegar, canned wild-caught salmon and sardines, avocado or coconut oil mayonnaise, and unsweetened ketchup

CONSIDER YOUR TOOLS

A few sharp knives of different sizes (think large for squash and small for avocados), a cutting board, and a few large mixing bowls are essential. You will also need some other items.

- **Storage:** Because plastic, and even BPA-free plastic, has known endocrine-disrupting chemicals (the ones that mimic estrogen, so endo suffers should always avoid them), it's important to stock up on glass or metal containers with secure lids. An assortment of Mason jars in several sizes works well, as do some draw-string canvas bags for easy veggie storage in the refrigerator.

- **Cooking gear:** You'll need a ceramic or cast iron pan ("no nonstick pans, please," said your endo), an assortment of baking sheets and dishes, as well as a big ol' pot. If you can swing it, consider an Instant Pot® to save time.

- **Food processor:** If you can make one investment in your kitchen, I recommend a food processor with both shredding and slicing attachments. This machine will become your sous chef, and boy can she chop, slice, and dice hours off your kitchen time. For a placeholder in the meantime, consider a handheld slicer called a mandoline.

TIDY YOUR KITCHEN

It sounds basic, but if you're constantly cooking in a cluttered kitchen it may start to stress you out. Get rid of gadgets and clutter, arrange your cabinets so you know where everything is, don't let things stack up, and always do a quick clean before and after a batch cook.

TRACK YOUR SYMPTOMS

When I was really sick I used to say "My body hates me." I seemed to have every symptom under the sun, and could not understand why. It was only when I diligently started tracking my symptoms that I began to see a pattern. Some symptoms were cyclical, some were exacerbated by food, and many were stress related. By understanding what were the triggers (and when to expect them), I felt like I had taken some control back in my life. It's something I have all my clients do as well.

That's why part of the four-week plan will be tracking how you're feeling in what I call a Food and Mood Journal. Tracking symptoms will not only help you learn to *listen* to your body, but also to better understand where symptoms are coming from, be they foods, activities, relationships, or job stressors.

I also recommend tracking everything—digestion, emotions, muscle aches—rather than just pelvic pain, so you can see the full picture of what's going on. This may be helpful when seeking reasons for flares, but is also a great long-term project to help you better see your healing trajectory. Because holistic healing is slow and steady, jotting down all your symptoms now will help you look back in six months to see just how far you've come without realizing it.

To help you, I've added a simple symptom tracker at the end of the book. Use this as a basic guide to jot down your symptoms so you can notice if anything intensifies or minimizes as you switch to the diet in this book. The more you get in touch with your body and listen to her, rather than hate her, the better off you'll be.

Five Troubleshooting Tips

Changing your routine, food culture, and diet is no easy feat! Use these five tips to help you on your way.

1. **Beginner chefs:** Do not aim for perfection, just chop, toss, cook, eat. This will get easier the more you practice. You will definitely ruin some recipes, and that's okay. You are not a failure—you're learning, and ruining some recipes is simply part of the process.

2. **Cravings:** If you end up craving junk food favorites, ask yourself what you're really after. Salt? Fat? Decadent? Challenge yourself to recreate that desire through whole foods rather than bingeing on packaged stuff.

3. **Digestion:** Digestive issues often crop up while changing your diet, not to mention the "carb flu," the temporarily sick feeling you may experience as you eliminate processed, refined grains and sugars. Increase whole foods and fiber slowly to avoid too many symptoms of going cold turkey, and always remember to chew and salivate to help digestion. Seriously, ladies, chew.

4. **More water overall, less at meals:** More fiber, more protein, more water! Aim to drink at least half your body weight in ounces (so if you weigh 130 pounds, drink 65 ounces or more). But not at meals, so your digestive system has less work to do.

5. **Focus on "good enough" over perfection:** It took me about two years to really understand the whole-foods lifestyle. Meaning? Be patient! Go slow! This is not a crash diet, it's a lifestyle swap, so make incremental changes that you can stick to. Learn to love whole foods and you'll never, ever regret it.

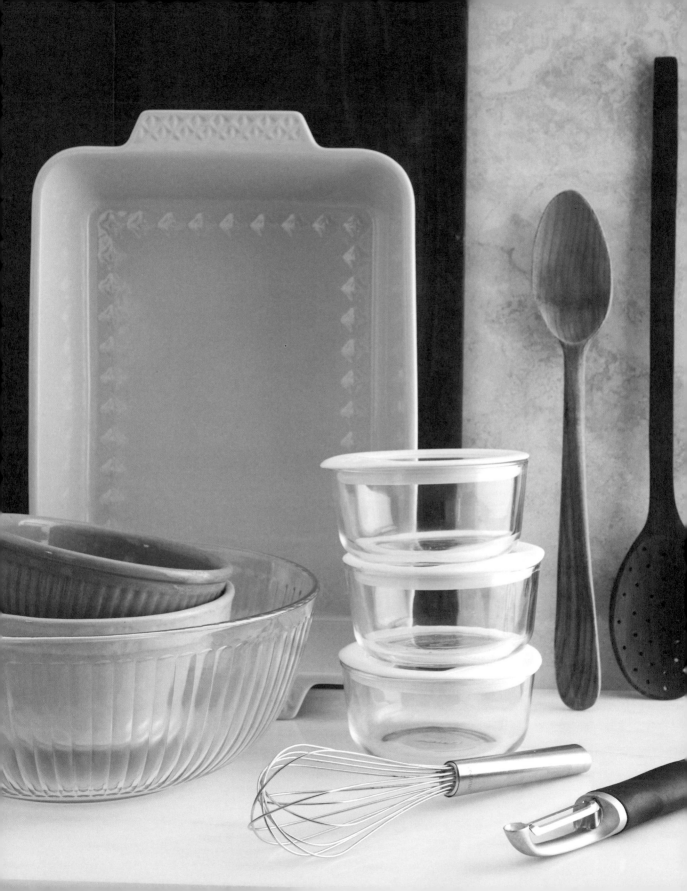

CHAPTER 5

The Meal Plan

The main emphasis of the meal plan is whole foods, yes, but just as important is the focus on batch cooking. Batch cooking means doubling or even tripling the recipe quantities so you can reheat the meal another day, or even freeze some for next week.

Learning this habit now will be the best thing you've ever done when you start spending time in the kitchen *really* cooking, since cleaning, chopping, cooking, and cleanup takes much more time than opening a box of cereal. Being a woman with chronic illness, saving time in the kitchen means saving energy for healing.

To help you, nearly all the baking recipes are set at 400°F so you can easily plan to bake numerous dishes at once. Also, this meal plan is not a low-FODMAP plan, so if you want to follow the low-FODMAP substitutions, please adjust accordingly!

Freezing Batch Cooking

Freezing leftovers in plastic freezer bags or containers is easiest, but best avoided due to their BPA content. Instead, consider heatproof glass containers such as Mason jars or Pyrex containers. Make sure to fill the glass containers only two-thirds full, to allow the contents to expand as they freeze and safely keep the glass from cracking.

WEEK 1

Your first week is dedicated to ensuring you eat a solid breakfast, your foundational meal of the day, to set your blood sugar up for success. You want to eat as much as you need (without fearing fat or calories) to make it three to five hours without needing more food. If balancing blood sugar is a concept you still don't get, just know a serious breakfast plus meal spacing are both needed to help start balancing blood sugar *now*.

PREP IT

I'm a big fan of making the majority of your weekday breakfasts on Sunday, so you don't have to think a second about it in the morning. This week you'll prep and make (that is, batch cook) *all* your breakfasts the Sunday before, and even freeze your Strawberries and Cream "Oatmeal" so you can defrost it Thursday night. Make time in your Sunday schedule, pop on your favorite podcast or music, and make it fun! You can, of course, make anything else in this book you like for other meals, but I mandate (in a nice way) that you focus on breakfast first and foremost this week. It's nonnegotiable.

SHOPPING LIST

Produce
Apples (3)
Collard greens (1 bunch)
Onions (2)
Spaghetti squash (1 medium)
Strawberries (3 cups)
Sweet potatoes (2)

Meat
Ground chicken or turkey, pastured
    (1.5 pounds)

Pantry items
Cinnamon
Coconut milk, full-fat (1 [12-ounce] can)
Coconut oil, organic
Extra-virgin olive oil, organic
Ground cloves
Ground turmeric
Raisins (1 bag; you'll use ⅓ cup this week)
Shredded coconut, unsweetened (1 bag;
    you'll need 1 cup this week)
Unrefined sea or Himalayan salt

WEEK ONE 7-DAY MEAL PLAN

Monday
   BREAKFAST: Moroccan Turkey and Sweet Potato Breakfast Bake (page 65)
   LUNCH: your choice
   DINNER: your choice

Tuesday
   BREAKFAST: Moroccan Turkey and Sweet Potato Breakfast Bake (page 65)
   LUNCH: your choice
   DINNER: your choice

Wednesday
   BREAKFAST: Moroccan Turkey and Sweet Potato Breakfast Bake (page 65)
   LUNCH: your choice
   DINNER: your choice

Thursday
   BREAKFAST: Moroccan Turkey and Sweet Potato Breakfast Bake (page 65)
   LUNCH: your choice
   DINNER: your choice

Friday
   BREAKFAST: Strawberries and Cream "Oatmeal" (page 69)
   LUNCH: your choice
   DINNER: your choice

Saturday
   BREAKFAST: Strawberries and Cream "Oatmeal" (page 69)
   LUNCH: your choice
   DINNER: your choice

Sunday
   BREAKFAST: Strawberries and Cream "Oatmeal" (page 69)
   LUNCH: your choice
   DINNER: your choice

WEEK 2

Your second week is going to build on your batch cooking skills to include all of your weekday lunches, plus one dinner. You'll even make enough Slow-Cooked Kalua Pork and Cabbage to freeze for next week. Keep up with your Funday (in other words, Sunday) batch cooking to set yourself up for success. Don't be overwhelmed about all the pantry items you bought for Week One; you'll be using them all for more recipes, so think of it as an investment.

PREP IT

On Sunday, batch cook Green Egg and Veggie Cups, Summer Herbed Carrots, and Hula Mashed Potatoes (cook all at 400°F for ease). While those are in the oven, put your Slow-Cooked Kalua Pork and Cabbage in your slow cooker or Instant Pot®, making sure to freeze half when it's done for next week. Tuesday night you'll make Broiled Maple Sesame Salmon and Asian Coleslaw Shreds for dinner, throwing the leftovers into Nori Wrap lunches for the following two days. Thursday night make your Bejeweled Breakfast Hash ahead of time for Friday through Sunday breakfasts. Saturday make a big pot of Bone Broth, which you'll freeze for next week. Are you starting to feel a little better with the extra veggie fiber, fats, and rainbow of nutrients?

SHOPPING LIST

Produce

Basil, fresh (⅔ cup)

Bell peppers, red (2)

Beets (3)

Broccoli (1 large; you'll need 2½ cups
   this week)

Brussels sprouts (4½ cups)

Carrots (12)

Cucumbers (2)

Fennel (1 bulb)

Garlic (1 bulb)

Kale (1 bunch)

Lemon (1 large)

Lime (1 large or 2 small)

Mango (1 large or 1 cup frozen)

Mint leaves, fresh (⅓ cup)

Onion (1)

Purple cabbage (1)

Rosemary, fresh (3 tablespoons)

Scallions (3)

Sweet potatoes (3)

Zucchini (2)

Meat and eggs

Bacon, organic (9 slices)

Beef knuckle bones (6, or 2 to 3 pounds of
   any bones)

Eggs, pastured (10)

Pork shoulder, 100-percent grass-fed
   (4 to 5 pounds)

Salmon fillet, wild-caught, skin-on (1)

Pantry items

Apple cider vinegar, raw (1 bottle;
   you'll need ⅓ cup this week)

Coconut aminos (1 bottle; you'll need
   ⅓ cup this week)

Coconut milk, full-fat (1 [12-ounce] can)

Cranberries, dried unsweetened
   (you'll need ⅓ cup this week)

Dijon mustard (you'll need 1 tablespoon
   this week)

Nori sheets (you'll need 6 this week)

Pecans (you'll need ¼ cup this week)

Salmon, wild-caught (3 [6-ounce] cans)

Sesame oil, organic (you'll need ⅓ cup
   this week)

Thai sweet chili sauce (you'll need
   3 tablespoons this week)

Dried herbs and spices

Basil

Garlic powder

Nutmeg

Onion powder

Red pepper, crushed

Thyme

WEEK TWO 7-DAY MEAL PLAN

Monday
BREAKFAST: Green Egg and Veggie Cups (page 63) + Summer Herbed Carrots (page 79)
LUNCH: Slow-Cooked Kalua Pork and Cabbage (page 113) + Hula Mashed Potatoes (page 89)
DINNER: your choice

Tuesday
BREAKFAST: Green Egg and Veggie Cups (page 63) + Hula Mashed Potatoes (page 89)
LUNCH: Slow-Cooked Kalua Pork and Cabbage (page 113) + Summer Herbed Carrots (page 79)
DINNER: Broiled Maple Sesame Salmon (page 95) + Asian Coleslaw Shreds (page 118)

Wednesday
BREAKFAST: Green Egg and Veggie Cups (page 63) + Hula Mashed Potatoes (page 89)
LUNCH: Nori Wraps (page 94) using leftover Broiled Maple Sesame Salmon (page 95)
+ Summer Herbed Carrots (page 79)
DINNER: your choice

Thursday
BREAKFAST: Green Egg and Veggie Cups (page 63) + Summer Herbed Carrots (page 79)
LUNCH: Nori Wraps (page 94) using leftover Broiled Maple Sesame Salmon (page 95)
+ Asian Coleslaw Shreds (page 118)
DINNER: your choice

Friday
BREAKFAST: Bejeweled Breakfast Hash (page 66)
LUNCH: Slow-Cooked Kalua Pork and Cabbage (page 113) + Asian Coleslaw Shreds (page 118)
DINNER: your choice

Saturday
BREAKFAST: Bejeweled Breakfast Hash (page 66)
LUNCH: your choice
DINNER: your choice

Sunday
BREAKFAST: Bejeweled Breakfast Hash (page 66)
LUNCH: your choice
DINNER: your choice

WEEK 3

You're on a roll! This week you'll focus on breakfasts, lunches, and dinners for your weekday fare, even making enough extras to freeze for next week (your next week self thanks you in advance). And don't worry, although it seems foreign at first, you'll start to get used to buying so much produce each week. It's what needs to happen so you know you're eating enough veggies, and this week you'll be eating up to 42g of fiber on some days.

PREP IT

On Sunday you'll spend about two to three hours making Sun Buns, Herbed Drumsticks, Baked Apples and Onions, and (six servings of) Greek Roasted Beets, while also prepping (chopping and cleaning) your veggies for your three Big Fat Green Smoothies this week. Notice how everything but the Sun Buns bakes at 400°F for ease? Monday night you'll make Meatloaf Muffins with Apples and Beets (make six servings to freeze half for next week), Caramelized Garden Tomatoes, and Cinnamon, Cacao, and Cayenne Cauliflower, eating the leftovers for breakfast and lunch. Also defrost three servings of Slow-Cooked Kalua Pork and Cabbage from last week. Wednesday defrost your Bone Broth for Egg Drop Soup for breakfast, and make Cocoa Beef Ragu with Spaghetti Squash Noodles (six servings to freeze half for next week) to round out your dinners. Friday night prep your chia for weekend breakfasts, and for the weekend throw together any leftovers for lunch or dinner so you can empty your refrigerator out for Week Four.

SHOPPING LIST

Produce

Apples (5)

Avocadoes (4)

Baby spinach (3 cups)

Bananas (2; peel and freeze these)

Beets (8)

Bell peppers, green (3)

Berries, mixed (1 cup)

Carrot (1)

Cauliflower (2 heads)

Cherry tomatoes (6 cups)

Cucumbers (2)

Lemon, large (1)

Mint leaves (⅓ cup)

Mushrooms (6 cups)

Onion, red (1)

Onions (3)

Scallions (2)

Spaghetti squash (1)

Tomatoes (3)

Zucchini (5)

Meat and eggs

Chicken drumsticks, pastured (1 pound)

Eggs, pastured (4)

Ground beef, 100-percent grass-fed
(5 pounds; remember, half of this is for
next week)

Smoked salmon, wild-caught (1 pound)

Pantry items

(You should already have shredded
coconut and dried cranberries
stocked)

Blackstrap molasses (1 bottle)

Cacao powder, raw

Chia seeds

Collagen powder, grass-fed (Vital
Proteins brand is great)

Coconut milk, full-fat (2 [12-ounce] cans)

Coconut yogurt, unsweetened (you'll
need ½ cup this week)

Crushed tomatoes (6 cups)

Tomato paste (1 [6-ounce] glass jar; you'll
need 6 tablespoons this week)

Walnuts, shelled (you'll need ¾ cup
this week)

Worcestershire sauce, gluten-free

Dried herbs and spices

Cayenne pepper

Italian seasoning mix

Oregano

WEEK THREE 7-DAY MEAL PLAN

Monday
BREAKFAST: Smoked Salmon on Sun Buns (page 61) + Big Fat Green Smoothie (page 60)
LUNCH: Herbed Drumsticks (page 104) + 2 servings Greek Roasted Beets (page 123)
DINNER: Meatloaf Muffins with Apples and Beets (page 108) + Cinnamon, Cacao, and Cayenne Cauliflower (page 82) + Caramelized Garden Tomatoes (page 73)

Tuesday
BREAKFAST: Smoked Salmon on Sun Buns (page 61) + Big Fat Green Smoothie (page 60)
LUNCH: Herbed Drumsticks (page 104) + 2 servings Greek Roasted Beets (page 123)
DINNER: Slow-Cooked Kalua Pork and Cabbage (page 113) + Baked Apples and Onions (page 88)

Wednesday
BREAKFAST: Smoked Salmon on Sun Buns (page 61) + Big Fat Green Smoothie (page 60)
LUNCH: Meatloaf Muffins with Apples and Beets (page 108) + 2 servings Cinnamon, Cacao, and Cayenne Cauliflower (page 82)
DINNER: Cocoa Beef Ragu (page 110) + Spaghetti Squash Noodles (page 86)

Thursday
BREAKFAST: Egg Drop Soup (page 62) with Sun Buns (page 122) + Caramelized Garden Tomatoes (page 73)
LUNCH: Herbed Drumsticks (page 104) + 2 servings Greek Roasted Beets (page 123)
DINNER: Slow-Cooked Kalua Pork and Cabbage (page 113) + Baked Apples and Onions (page 88)

Friday
BREAKFAST: Egg Drop Soup (page 62) with Sun Buns (page 122) + Caramelized Garden Tomatoes (page 73)
LUNCH: Meatloaf Muffins with Apples and Beets (page 108) + 2 servings Cinnamon, Cacao, and Cayenne Cauliflower (page 82)
DINNER: Cocoa Beef Ragu (page 110) + Spaghetti Squash Noodles (page 86)

Saturday
BREAKFAST: Coco-Carrot Chia with Berries (page 68)
LUNCH: leftovers
DINNER: Cocoa Beef Ragu (page 110) + Spaghetti Squash Noodles (page 86)

Sunday
BREAKFAST: Coco-Carrot Chia with Berries (page 68)
LUNCH: leftovers
DINNER: leftovers

WEEK 4

By now your pantry should be well stocked with fats and flavors to make your whole foods taste exceptional, and you should (hopefully) be starting to feel a little better by eating much less sugar, starches, and potentially inflammatory triggers. (You should already have the raisins, cacao powder, apple cider vinegar, coconut aminos, Dijon mustard, olive oil, sesame oil, and molasses.) This week you're going to go for the gold: three square meals that will each day meet or exceed your RDA for vitamins and minerals (in some cases double or triple—not kidding), averaging around 100 net carbs per day, and hitting between 30g and 41g of fiber per day!

PREP IT

On Sunday spend a solid three hours making the Huevos Deliciosos con Salsa (you will add the salsa fresh before serving), Offally Good Sausage (freeze for Thursday), I Can't Believe I'm Eating Sardine Salad, Chopped Green Salad, Fertility Goddess Dressing, Roasted Fennel, and Golden Hour Fish Pie. Again, all the oven recipes are baked at 400°F for ease, so don't be overwhelmed. Tuesday evening you'll make Turkey Burgers with Cashew Cheese and Hippie Collard Greens, and remember to defrost your Meatloaf Muffins with Apples and Beets from last week for lunch tomorrow. Wednesday night you'll prep the rest of your breakfasts and weekday lunches by making Sweet Sesame Mushrooms and Greens, defrosting your Offally Good Sausages and Meatloaf Muffins with Apples and Beets, and prepping your Speedy Salads. Friday defrost your Cocoa Beef Ragu from last week to fill your Ragu-Stuffed Bell Peppers for weekend lunches, and Saturday night you'll make Thai Shrimp Scampi and Broccoli Fried "Rice" for your weekend dinners. Before you go to bed each night, make a quart of Nettle Tea Blood Infusion for the next day, and leave it to steep overnight.

SHOPPING LIST

Produce
Apples, green (2)
Avocados (3)
Baby spinach (1 cup)
Basil leaves (¼ cup)
Bell peppers, red (6)
Bok choy (about 3 large heads; 16 cups)
Carrots (6)
Cauliflower (1 head)
Celery (1 head)
Cherry tomatoes (3 cups)
Collard greens (about 2 bunches; 2 pounds)
Cucumber (2)
Fennel (2 bulbs)
Leeks (2)
Mushrooms (8 cups)
Onion, red (1)
Onions (3)
Parsley (1 bunch)
Plantains, yellow (3)
Romaine lettuce (1 head)
Salad mix (10 cups)
Scallions (1 to 2 bunches; 8 pieces)
Tarragon (1 bunch)
Zucchini (3)

Meat and eggs
Beef liver, 100-percent grass-fed
    (4 ounces; come on, I dare you)
Cod (1 pound)
Eggs, pastured (11)
Ground beef, 100-percent grass-fed
    (1 pound)

Ground turkey, pastured (½ pound)
Bacon, organic (5 slices)
Shrimp (1 pound)

Pantry items
Avocado oil- or coconut oil-based
    mayonnaise (3 tablespoons)
Cashews, raw (2 cups)
Coconut milk, full-fat (1 [12-ounce] can)
    (you will need 2 tablespoons this week)
Crushed tomatoes (1 cup)
Honey, raw (2 tablespoons)
Nettle tea (4 cups; look on moun-
    tainroseherbs.com to buy in bulk)
Pistachios, shelled (1 cup)
Red raspberry leaf tea (4 cups)
Salmon, wild-caught (2 [6-ounce] cans)
Salsa, organic (1½ cups)
Sardines, wild-caught (1 [4-ounce] can)
Sesame seeds (2 tablespoons)
Sweet chili sauce (2 tablespoons)
Tahini (1 [12-ounce] jar; you will need
    ½ cup this week)
Tomato paste (3 tablespoons)

Dried herbs and spices
Bay leaves
Black pepper
Chili powder
Ground ginger
Sage
Nutritional yeast

WEEK FOUR 7-DAY MEAL PLAN

Monday

BREAKFAST: Huevos Deliciosos con Salsa (page 64)

LUNCH: Chopped Green Salad (page 117) + I Can't Believe I'm Eating Sardine Salad (page 92) with Fertility Goddess Dressing (page 142)

AFTERNOON PICK-ME-UP: Nettle Tea Blood Infusion (page 129)

DINNER: Golden Hour Fish Pie (page 101) + Roasted Fennel (page 74)

Tuesday

BREAKFAST: Huevos Deliciosos con Salsa (page 64)

LUNCH: Chopped Green Salad (page 117) + I Can't Believe I'm Eating Sardine Salad (page 92) with Fertility Goddess Dressing (page 142)

AFTERNOON PICK-ME-UP: Nettle Tea Blood Infusion (page 129)

DINNER: Turkey Burgers with Cashew Cheese (page 107) + Hippie Collard Greens (page 78)

Wednesday

BREAKFAST: Huevos Deliciosos con Salsa (page 64)

LUNCH: Meatloaf Muffins with Apples and Beets (defrosted) (page 108) + Speedy Salad (page 116) with Fertility Goddess Dressing (page 142)

AFTERNOON PICK-ME-UP: Nettle Tea Blood Infusion (page 129)

DINNER: Golden Hour Fish Pie (page 101) + Roasted Fennel (page 74)

Thursday

BREAKFAST: Offally Good Sausage (page 67) + Sweet Sesame Mushrooms and Greens (page 85)

LUNCH: Chopped Green Salad (page 117) + I Can't Believe I'm Eating Sardine Salad (page 92) with Fertility Goddess Dressing (page 142)

AFTERNOON PICK-ME-UP: Nettle Tea Blood Infusion (page 129)

DINNER: Turkey Burgers with Cashew Cheese (page 107) + Hippie Collard Greens (page 78)

Friday

BREAKFAST: Offally Good Sausage (page 67) + Sweet Sesame Mushrooms and Greens (page 85)

LUNCH: Meatloaf Muffins with Apples and Beets (page 108) + Speedy Salad (page 116) with Fertility Goddess Dressing (page 142)

AFTERNOON PICK-ME-UP: Nettle Tea Blood Infusion (page 129)

DINNER: Golden Hour Fish Pie (page 101) + Roasted Fennel (page 74)

Saturday

BREAKFAST: Offally Good Sausage (page 67) + Sweet Sesame Mushrooms and Greens (page 85)

LUNCH: Ragu-Stuffed Bell Peppers (page 111) (part defrosted) + Cashew Cheese (page 145)

AFTERNOON PICK-ME-UP: Nettle Tea Blood Infusion (page 129)

DINNER: Thai Shrimp Scampi (page 98) + Broccoli Fried "Rice" (page 81)

Sunday

BREAKFAST: Offally Good Sausage (page 67) + Sweet Sesame Mushrooms and Greens (page 85)

LUNCH: Ragu-Stuffed Bell Peppers (page 111) (part defrosted) + Cashew Cheese (page 145)

AFTERNOON PICK-ME-UP: Nettle Tea Blood Infusion (page 129)

DINNER: Thai Shrimp Scampi (page 98) + Broccoli Fried "Rice" (page 81)

If Your Symptoms Persist

If after adopting a whole-foods, veggie-abundant, nutrient-dense diet like this you still don't feel well, please don't think you're a lost cause! As I mentioned at the beginning of this book, you may have some gut infections, a specific intolerance, or leaky gut, all of which could make you feel lousy unless you try a specific elimination diet—which I wholeheartedly recommend—based on your symptoms.

If after applying the program in this book you feel worse in terms of bloating (like, you're a bloatation station) or bowel issues, consider a strict low-FODMAP diet for two to four weeks to see if you notice improvements. If you do, I recommend working with a functional health practitioner to find out why you're reacting, and help you reverse this trend so you can eat those healthy foods again.

If, on the other hand, you still have lots of symptoms, your own body may truly be reacting to certain healthy foods. As I mentioned, diets like the Paleo Autoimmune Protocol Diet remove all the big triggers, including eggs, dairy, grains, nightshades, soy, legumes, caffeine, and sugar. So if you react to any of these foods you may need a 30- to 90-day serious elimination gut reset to really start addressing this issue.

The takeaway is this: Don't stress if you're not "fixed." The goal of this book is to lay out a general foundation of how to eat (tons of veggies, plus quality meats, fats, fruit), and you, dear reader, may just need extra TLC to get where you need to be.

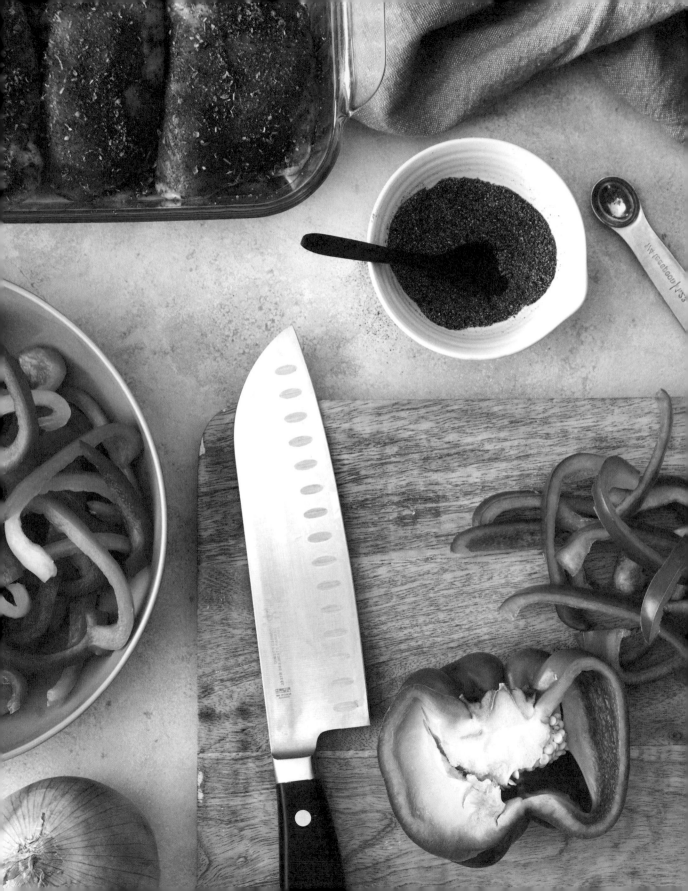

PART III

The Recipes

And finally to the meat of the book (pun intended), the recipes! Here you will find 75 delicious options to fill your nutrient quotas while keeping your taste buds happy. A friendly reminder that quality food procurement is an important feature of whole-foods cooking, for nutrient density, animal welfare, and toxin avoidance. Aim to buy all produce as organic and local as possible. As for animal products, I recommend all eggs be pastured or at least free-range and organic, meat and poultry be 100-percent grass-fed or pastured, fish be wild-caught, and your salt be unrefined sea salt or Himalayan salt so that you're consuming a rainbow of minerals from this seasoning, rather than highly refined, sodium-only table salt. If you're budgeting, at least follow the Dirty Dozen™ rule for produce (see page 154) and simply do the best you can with animal products. Additionally, avoid buying things like tomato paste, sauces, and condiments in plastic containers or aluminum cans (which are lined with plastics), since plastics are known endocrine disruptors that make your endo quite unhappy. Simply look for glass instead. Most importantly, have fun!

Smoked Salmon on Sun Buns, Page 61

CHAPTER 6

Breakfasts

Big Fat Green Smoothie

Prep time: 10 minutes · ***Serves:*** 1

30 MINUTE | LOW FODMAP | NUT FREE

Smoothies aren't my favorite breakfast food, mostly because they don't fill you up for longer than a few hours. However, this one will do a lot better: Rich in veggies, low in sugar, high in fat and protein, and super duper delicious. This smoothie has 12 grams of veggie-based fiber (more than some people get all day), tons of minerals, B vitamins, and healthy fats.

1 cup spinach

½ ripe avocado

½ zucchini

½ cucumber

½ frozen banana

Juice of ½ lemon

2 tablespoons grass-fed collagen powder

½ cup full-fat coconut milk

½ cup water

¼ to ½ teaspoon cinnamon

1. Roughly chop the spinach, avocado, zucchini, cucumber, and banana.

2. Put all the ingredients in the blender. Purée, adding filtered water to thin as desired.

POWER BOOST: Smoothies are a great way to toss in extras for a health boost. Consider adding fresh turmeric, ginger, spirulina, or a whole food source of vitamin C for extra anti-inflammatory power. Add one or two egg yolks for a fertility boost.

LOW FODMAP: Use only ⅛ of an avocado.

PER SERVING Calories: 581; Saturated Fat: 28g; Total Fat: 43g; Protein: 22g; Total Carbs: 38g; Fiber: 13g; Sodium: 157mg

Smoked Salmon on Sun Buns

Prep time: 10 minutes · *Serves:* 2

30 MINUTE | LOW FODMAP

Wild-caught salmon should be an endo staple because it's high in omega-3 fats—a nutrient we're often severely lacking—which help quell inflammation. Smoked salmon is also great for breakfast because it's fast, easy, and will really fill you up. Remember to add a few cups of veggies on the side to make this a well rounded meal. Or pair it with Sweet Sesame Mushrooms and Greens (page 85), Caramelized Garden Tomatoes (page 73), or Rainbow Unicorn Carrot and Beet Shreds (page 80).

2 Sun Buns (page 122)

6 to 8 ounces wild-caught smoked salmon

1 avocado, sliced

1 tomato, sliced

Sea salt

Freshly ground black pepper

Green Herb Oil (page 140) (optional)

1. Toast the Sun Buns.
2. Top with smoked salmon, avocado, tomato, salt, pepper, and Green Herb Oil, if using.

LOW FODMAP: Use only ⅛ of an avocado.

PER SERVING Calories: 479; Saturated Fat: 5g; Total Fat: 26g; Protein: 25g; Total Carbs: 41g; Fiber: 17g; Sodium: 983mg

Egg Drop Soup

Prep time: 5 minutes · *Cook time:* 5 minutes · *Serves:* 2

30 MINUTE | LOW FODMAP | NUT FREE

If you have bone broth on hand, you can make this Egg Drop Soup in a jiffy. It's über satisfying, and pairs well with whatever veggies you throw on the side. Pair with Broccoli Fried "Rice" (page 81), Nori Crisps (page 119), Perfect Stir-Fry (page 84), or Eggplant Rounds (page 76) to get your veggies in. This healing soup is great for pre- or post-surgery, prenatal, or postpartum. Heck, bone broth–based soup is great any time if you have endo.

4 cups Bone Broth (page 148)

4 eggs

Sea salt

2 scallions, chopped (optional)

Red pepper flakes (optional)

Fish sauce (optional)

1. In a large pot, heat the bone broth to a low simmer.
2. While the broth is heating, crack and scramble the eggs in a medium bowl.
3. When the broth reaches a low simmer, turn off the heat. Use a large spoon to swirl the broth while you slowly add in the egg mixture. The egg should cook on contact with the broth, even though the heat is off. The eggs should form soft ribbons, rather than lumps.
4. Top with scallions, red pepper flakes, and a few dashes of fish sauce if you like.

SUBS AND SWAPS: If you don't tolerate eggs you can always quick chop some sausage and veggies, sauté until lightly cooked, and add to the bone broth for a quick breakfast soup. This need not be fancy.

PER SERVING Calories: 254; Saturated Fat: 7g; Total Fat: 17g; Protein: 23g; Total Carbs: 3g; Fiber: 0g; Sodium: 418mg

Green Egg and Veggie Cups

Prep time: 10 minutes · ***Cook time:*** 12 minutes · ***Serves:*** 4

30 MINUTE | LOW FODMAP | NUT FREE | VEGETARIAN

Frittatas are one of the easiest make-ahead breakfasts and they multitask as a quick snack if you're crashing. Cook them in a muffin tin with phytonutrient-rich herbs and they're even better. Each cup provides essential amino acids and fertility-boosting nutrients like choline, vitamins A and D, and hormone supporting cholesterol, plus veggie-based fiber. Mix it up and use any veggies or herbs you want; the basic is that each cup should be half veggies and half green eggs. If you tolerate eggs, these are incredible nutrient bombs. If you like goat cheese, that tastes great on top.

Coconut oil

1 cup shredded or finely diced broccoli

1 cup shredded or finely diced zucchini

1 green bell pepper, seeded and shredded, or finely diced

8 eggs

¼ teaspoon unrefined sea salt

½ cup packed fresh basil

1. Preheat the oven to 400°F and grease a 12-cup muffin tray with coconut oil.

2. Evenly portion out the shredded veggie mixture into the muffin cups.

3. Put the eggs, salt, and basil in a blender and pulse until blended. Pour the green egg mixture on top of the veggies. If you have leftovers you can make extra muffins or simply scramble the eggs for breakfast (or save them for tomorrow).

4. Bake for 12 to 14 minutes. Give the pan a shake to see if they're done. The eggs are done when the middle of the "cupcake" is just set (it doesn't wobble like Jell-O).

MAKE IT FAST: Grab any leftovers from the refrigerator, such as fajita veggies, roasted tomatoes, or sautéed mushrooms and greens. Spoon some into greased muffin pans, scramble an egg into each, and bake for 12 to 14 minutes at 400°F.

PER SERVING Calories: 154; Saturated Fat: 4g; Total Fat: 10g; Protein: 12g; Total Carbs: 5g; Fiber: 1g; Sodium: 158mg

Huevos Deliciosos con Salsa

Prep time: 20 minutes · **Cook time:** 30 minutes · **Serves:** 4

NUT FREE

When I went to school in Santa Barbara, California, I was obsessed with huevos rancheros burritos. Going gluten free and lower carb meant I had to say goodbye to the flour wrap and chunky potatoes, but luckily I realized I could replace them with so much more flavor. This is a nutrient-dense breakfast that will keep you running for hours. Use your food processor to quickly slice the onions and peppers. Garnish with cilantro and jalapeño peppers and serve with a side salad.

Extra-virgin olive oil

1 onion, thinly sliced

2 bell peppers, seeded and thinly sliced

2 plantains, peeled and diced

2 tablespoons tomato paste

2 cups cherry tomatoes, halved

1 cup Bone Broth (page 148)

1 cup salsa

½ teaspoon sea salt

1 teaspoon dried oregano

½ teaspoon garlic powder

1 tablespoon chili powder

8 eggs

1. Preheat the oven to 400°F.

2. In a large skillet on the stovetop, heat a little oil over medium heat. Add the onion and bell peppers and cook until they just start to turn golden brown, about 5 minutes. Add the plantains and sauté for 2 more minutes. Stir in the tomato paste, tomatoes, bone broth, salsa, salt, oregano, garlic powder, and chili powder. Simmer uncovered until thickened, about 10 minutes.

3. If you're cooking in an ovenproof skillet, crack the eggs into the sauce and put the whole thing in the oven. Otherwise, transfer the mixture to a baking dish, then crack in the eggs.

4. Bake until set (not Jell-O-like), for 13 to 15 minutes.

SUBS AND SWAPS: If you don't tolerate eggs, you can easily top this with precooked Offally Good Sausage (page 67), or chicken from the Chicken Fajitas Bowl (page 105) instead.

LOW FODMAP: Leave out the onions and garlic powder.

PER SERVING Calories: 333; Saturated Fat: 3g; Total Fat: 11g; Protein: 19g; Total Carbs: 47g; Fiber: 7g; Sodium: 725mg

Moroccan Turkey and Sweet Potato Breakfast Bake

Prep time: 10 minutes · *Cook time:* 40 to 50 minutes · *Serves:* 3 to 4

NUT FREE

This is a nice stepping stone breakfast for women ready to balance their blood sugar, but are a little uncertain about eating a big, solid breakfast first thing in the morning. Chicken and turkey are lighter protein options and, when paired with apples and sweet potato, offer a sweet and savory middle ground many women can approve of. Make ahead for ease, and eat as much as you need to feel full until lunch!

1 to 2 tablespoons coconut oil

1 onion, chopped

1 pound ground turkey or chicken

2 cups collard greens or other farmers' market greens, stemmed and shredded

1 teaspoon sea salt

2 teaspoons cinnamon

½ teaspoon turmeric

¼ teaspoon ground cloves

1 large sweet potato, peeled and chopped into 1-inch chunks

1 apple, cored and chopped into 1-inch chunks

3 tablespoons raisins

1. Preheat the oven to 400°F.

2. In a large skillet over medium heat, heat the coconut oil. Add the onion and cook until it's golden and translucent, 5 to 8 minutes. Add the ground turkey, collard greens, salt, cinnamon, turmeric, and cloves. Cook until browned.

3. In the skillet, add the apple and raisins and toss together with the sweet potato. Pour the mixture into a baking dish.

4. Cover the dish with aluminum foil and bake for 35 to 45 minutes, or until the sweet potato is tender.

LOW FODMAP: Instead of the onion and apple, use eggplant, fennel, or zucchini.

MAKE IT FAST: Make this a quick skillet by quickly browning the meat, then adding in precooked sweet potato or winter squash and Baked Apples and Onions (page 88).

PER SERVING Calories: 298; Saturated Fat: 1g; Total Fat: 4g; Protein: 38g; Total Carbs: 32g; Fiber: 6g; Sodium: 733mg

Bejeweled Breakfast Hash

Prep time: 20 minutes · *Cook time:* 25 minutes · *Serves:* 4 to 6

NUT FREE

This breakfast is not only beautiful with its jewel-colored veggies, but is great for starting your day since it has all the nutrients you'll need for a busy morning. Plus, you can make it ahead, so it's fab for on-the-goers. Beets are great for liver support, yams are full of the phytonutrient beta-carotene, Brussels sprouts support estrogen detoxification, and bacon makes everything taste so *ono* (Hawaiian for delicious).

8 bacon slices

1 large yam, cubed (peeled only if you prefer)

2 cups cubed beets (peeled only if you prefer)

3 cups halved Brussels sprouts

1 teaspoon dried rosemary

¼ teaspoon sea salt

½ teaspoon garlic powder

½ teaspoon onion powder

¼ cup unsweetened dried cranberries

1. Preheat the oven to 400°F.

2. Cook the bacon in a large pan until crispy (even if you like it soft, crispy bacon works best for this recipe). Remove the bacon from the pan and set it aside on a paper towel.

3. In a large mixing bowl, add the yam, beets, and Brussels sprouts. Pour the bacon grease from the pan over them and carefully toss to coat. Then stir in the rosemary, salt, garlic powder, and onion powder and toss to coat.

4. Spread the veggies on a large baking sheet; take care that they are not stacked on top of one other, which will steam them rather than roast them. Place the pan in the oven and roast for 20 to 25 minutes, until the veggies are tender on the inside and crisp on the outside.

5. Portion out 4 to 6 servings, mixing in the dried cranberries and crumbling the bacon on top as you go.

SUBS AND SWAPS: Switch out the veggies listed here for any of your hearty faves, such as broccoli, cauliflower, or winter squash.

LEFTOVERS AND EXTRAS: If you batch cook this recipe and prefer to keep your bacon crispy, save it in a separate container so it doesn't absorb extra moisture from the veggies.

PER SERVING Calories: 317; Saturated Fat: 5g; Total Fat: 16g; Protein: 18g; Total Carbs: 26g; Fiber: 7g; Sodium: 949mg

Offally Good Sausage and Farmers Breakfast

Prep time: 20 minutes · ***Cook time:*** 10 minutes · ***Serves:*** 4

NUT FREE

Offal is a word for organ meats. It's pronounced "awful," which I am sure is based on its awfully delicious flavor. Seriously, you won't even know there is organ meat in these sausages; they taste so good! Proportions and spices are everything. I promise, not even your kids will know there's an offal-lot of nutrition inside. Eat one to two sausages with 2 to 3 cups of veggies of your choice for what I call a farmers breakfast. It's a meal that will fill up your nutrient tanks and balance your blood sugar for hours. I eat this nearly every day, and know you'll like it too.

¼ pound beef liver

1 pound grass-fed ground beef

½ teaspoon garlic powder

½ teaspoon onion powder

½ teaspoon dried oregano

½ teaspoon cinnamon

½ teaspoon turmeric

½ teaspoon sea salt (or less if you're adding bacon)

4 bacon slices, roughly chopped (optional)

Coconut oil

1. Grind the liver—be brave! You can cut the liver into strips, freeze it, and grate the frozen strips with a box grater or food processor. Or, if you have a high-powered blender, you don't have to freeze it. Just cut it into chunks and process it until it's puréed.

2. In a large bowl, mix the ground liver and ground beef with the garlic powder, onion powder, oregano, cinnamon, turmeric, and salt. Bacon adds lots of additional yummy flavor, if you're using it. (If you're super scared of liver, just start with 2 tablespoons and work your way up. I swear, it won't kill you!)

3. Process all the ingredients in a food processor until blended smooth. Form the meat mixture into small sausage patties.

4. In a medium skillet, heat a layer of coconut oil. Add the sausage patties and fry for about 5 minutes on each side, until the patties are cooked through.

LEFTOVERS AND EXTRAS: These sausages will keep in the refrigerator for three to four days, or freeze the extras.

LOW FODMAP: Leave out the garlic and onion powders.

PER SERVING Calories: 247; Saturated Fat: 5g; Total Fat: 13g; Protein: 29g; Total Carbs: 2g; Fiber: 0g; Sodium: 329mg

Sunday Special #1:
Coco-Carrot Chia with Berries

Prep time: 15 minutes • ***Serves:*** 2

30 MINUTE | NUT FREE | LOW FODMAP

I call these sweeter breakfasts Sunday Specials because I want you to reserve them for a weekend treat, rather than for every day. Still, this breakfast packs a punch with fiber, veggies, berries, protein, iron-rich molasses, and full-fat coconut milk, all of which should help you last. Make it the night before, so the flavors have time to blend.

1 cup full-fat coconut milk

2 teaspoons blackstrap molasses

Pinch sea salt

¼ teaspoon cinnamon

2 tablespoons grass-fed collagen powder

¼ cup chia seeds

1 large carrot, shredded

2 tablespoons shredded unsweetened coconut

1 cup berries

1. Whisk together the coconut milk, molasses, salt, cinnamon, collagen, and chia seeds. Let sit for at least 15 minutes, or overnight in the refrigerator.

2. When the chia has absorbed the liquid and formed a pudding, mix in the carrot, coconut, and berries. Add more coconut milk if you want it a little less thick.

SUBS AND SWAPS: Swap zucchini or yacón (a tasty tuber) for the carrots. Switch papaya, apples, or any other local in-season fruit for the berries.

PER SERVING Calories: 517; Saturated Fat: 28g; Total Fat: 39g; Protein: 15g; Total Carbs: 34g; Fiber: 15g; Sodium: 214mg

Sunday Special #2:
Strawberries and Cream "Oatmeal"

Prep time: 10 minutes · *Cook time:* 10 minutes · *Serves:* 2

30 MINUTE | NUT FREE | LOW FODMAP

Many women have a hard time leaving their oatmeal behind when going grain-free—until they realize there's a delicious, low-carb replacement waiting for them. This is breakfast comfort food at its finest—warm and filling—and you may not miss your oatmeal after all. Because of the sweetness and heavy carb load of this breakfast, I hope you reserve it for a weekend treat.

2 cups cooked spaghetti squash

1 cup full-fat coconut milk

¾ cup shredded unsweetened coconut

2 cups sliced strawberries

Pinch sea salt

4 tablespoons grass-fed collagen powder

Raw honey or pure maple syrup (optional)

Nut Mylk Any Way (page 131) (optional)

1. If you don't have precooked spaghetti squash on hand (which I hope you do because you've been batch cooking), then prepare the squash as described on page 86.

2. Put the cooked squash in a food processor or blender and pulse/blend it with the coconut milk and shredded coconut, until it forms a slightly chunky oatmeal consistency.

3. In a medium pot, add the strawberries, salt, and collagen. Simmer uncovered on low heat for about 10 minutes, until it has thickened and the coconut is soft. You can simmer longer to thicken, if you desire.

4. Serve immediately, with a *moderate amount* of honey or maple syrup, and a touch of Nut Mylk Any Way (page 131), if you prefer.

LEFTOVERS AND EXTRAS: You can make enough in bulk for two to three days and keep it in the refrigerator. Reheat for breakfasts, which makes it Instant "Oatmeal" breakfast. Easy.

SUBS AND SWAPS: Exchange low-FODMAP spaghetti squash for sweet potatoes, yams, or plantains. Swap out strawberries for any other fruit. The basic recipe is the same.

PER SERVING Calories: 516; Saturated Fat: 34g; Total Fat: 40g; Protein: 19g; Total Carbs: 29g; Fiber: 8g; Sodium: 250mg

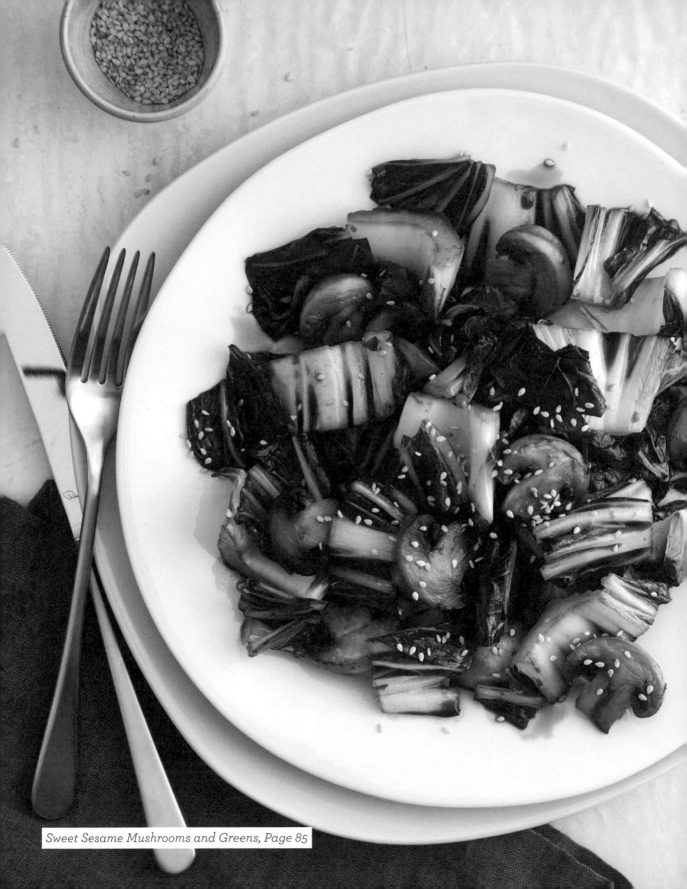

Sweet Sesame Mushrooms and Greens, Page 85

Plants

Green Bean Frites

Prep time: 10 minutes · *Cook time:* 20 minutes · *Serves:* 4

30 MINUTES | VEGAN

Although there's no true substitute for French fries, these rich and salty frites are an excellent stand-in. Green beans are an awesome low-starch vegetable, rich in antioxidant and anti-inflammatory properties and folate, and may help reduce the effect of cell-damaging free radicals, while olive oil and almonds are rich in polyphenols and vitamin E. Serve with Turkey Burgers (page 107) or Herbed Drumsticks (page 104) to make it a meal.

4 cups green beans, trimmed and very dry
Extra-virgin olive oil
½ teaspoon sea salt, divided
½ cup almond flour
½ teaspoon paprika
½ teaspoon garlic powder
½ teaspoon onion powder

1. Preheat the oven to 400°F.
2. In a large bowl, toss the green beans in oil to coat well, and place them on a baking sheet. Don't stack the beans on top of one another if you want them to be crisp—if you do, they'll steam. Sprinkle the green beans with ¼ teaspoon salt. Roast for 12 minutes.
3. While the beans are roasting, mix the almond flour, paprika, garlic powder, onion powder, and the remaining ¼ teaspoon salt in a small bowl.
4. After 12 minutes, shake the baking sheet to turn the beans, and dust them with the almond flour mixture. Return the pan to the oven and cook for 3 to 5 minutes more, for the coating to crisp up.

SUBS AND SWAPS: My favorite swap is kohlrabi! Peel and cut it into fries, season, and cook exactly the same way.

LOW FODMAP: Substitute 1 teaspoon of orange zest for the onion and garlic powder.

PER SERVING Calories: 96; Saturated Fat: 0g; Total Fat: 5g; Protein: 4g; Total Carbs: 11g; Fiber: 5g; Sodium: 244mg

Caramelized Garden Tomatoes

Prep time: 5 minutes · *Cook time:* 45 minutes · *Serves:* 2

LOW FODMAP | NUT FREE | VEGAN

If you've grown cherry tomatoes, you understand how you can suddenly have a glut (and if you haven't grown them before, now's the time to try!). What to do? Roast them. Cherry tomatoes are jam-packed with nutrients, and when roasted develop a deep, rich, and slightly sweet flavor reminiscent of Tuscany. Serve with Spaghetti Squash Noodles (page 86), or Lamb Meatballs with Minted Tahini Sauce (page 112) and a Speedy Salad (page 116).

2 pints cherry tomatoes

1 to 2 tablespoons extra-virgin olive oil

½ teaspoon sea salt

1. Preheat the oven to 400°F.
2. Put the tomatoes in a large bowl, add the oil, and toss to coat.
3. Place the tomatoes on a large baking sheet and sprinkle with salt. Bake for about 45 minutes, stirring halfway through, until the skins have shriveled or slightly split.
4. Enjoy hot, at room temperature, or chilled.

POWER BOOST: Top with Green Herb Oil (page 140).

PER SERVING Calories: 75; Saturated Fat: 0g; Total Fat: 2g; Protein: 3g; Total Carbs: 14g; Fiber: 4g; Sodium: 486mg

Roasted Fennel

Prep time: 10 minutes · *Cook time:* 40 minutes · *Serves:* 4

LOW FODMAP | NUT FREE | VEGAN

Fennel is perhaps the most underrated veggie I know. It's stunningly delicious, tender yet crunchy, and full of vitamin C, minerals, fiber, and phytonutrients. Plus, it aids digestion, which is a win-win for any tender endo-bellies. Raw fennel has a delicate licorice flavor that disappears when roasted, baking into a rich, caramelized veggie anyone can love.

2 large fennel bulbs, or 4 small

Extra-virgin olive oil

Sea salt

Balsamic vinegar reduction (optional)

1. Preheat the oven to 400°F.
2. Cut off the fennel fronds (save for salads if you like) and remove the outer leaves if they're woody or dry. Cut the bulbs into ½-inch slices.
3. Place the fronds on a roasting tray and drizzle with enough oil to coat. Sprinkle with salt.
4. Roast for 30 to 40 minutes, flipping halfway through to prevent one side from getting tougher than the other (this is important, or one side will definitely be tougher). The fennel is done when the edges are browning and caramelized.
5. Top with a balsamic vinegar reduction, if you like.

LEFTOVERS AND EXTRAS: Fennel is great hot or cold! Serve immediately as a hot side dish, reheat for tomorrow, or use chilled leftovers to top a salad.

PER SERVING Calories: 64; Saturated Fat: 0g; Total Fat: 2g; Protein: 2g; Total Carbs: 13g; Fiber: 5g; Sodium: 208mg

Zesty Zucchini

Prep time: 10 minutes · *Cook time:* 5 minutes · *Serves:* 4

30 MINUTES | LOW FODMAP | VEGAN

Zucchini is a great source of beta-carotene, vitamin C, potassium, and fiber, and is a fantastic low-starch food. To keep zucchini from being a soggy mess, cook quickly over high heat, and make sure to add plenty of salt and fat to your liking so you never think of zucchini as bland again. Just omit the pine nuts if they're a problem for you. To make it a meal, serve with Cocoa Beef Ragu (page 110) and Spaghetti Squash Noodles (page 86), or Chopped Green Salad (page 117) and Salmon Burgers (page 93).

4 medium zucchini, halved lengthwise

¼ teaspoon sea salt

1 to 2 tablespoons extra-virgin olive oil

½ cup toasted pine nuts

3 tablespoons finely minced fresh mint leaves

2 teaspoons lemon zest

1. Slice the zucchini into thick, half-moon slices, and lightly salt.

2. In a large skillet, heat the oil over medium-high heat. When the oil is hot, add the zucchini. Sauté until it is light golden brown but still slightly crisp (there's nothing worse than soggy zucchini!), for 4 to 5 minutes.

3. Remove the zucchini from the skillet and sprinkle with the pine nuts, mint, and lemon zest, plus more salt if you prefer. Serve immediately.

SUBS AND SWAPS: If you want simple roast zucchini, just omit the toppings. Easy!

PER SERVING Calories: 157; Saturated Fat: 1g; Total Fat: 13g; Protein: 5g; Total Carbs: 9g; Fiber: 3g; Sodium: 138mg

Eggplant Rounds

Prep time: 5 minutes · *Cook time:* 15 minutes · *Serves:* 4

30 MINUTES | NUT FREE | VEGAN

Eggplant is a finicky vegetable that can quickly wear out its welcome with its mushy ways. Yet, when cooked correctly, these gals are not only exquisitely tasty, but also full of potassium, magnesium, calcium, phosphorous, and tons of antioxidants. These rounds can be eaten as a side, or substituted in for a low-carb bun or mini taco. You can load eggplant rounds with toppings or dips, or add them to other dishes. Serve with Ragu-Stuffed Bell Peppers (page 111) and Caramelized Garden Tomatoes (page 73), or top a few rounds with smoked salmon or leftover chicken fajitas for a complete meal.

2 Italian eggplants

Extra-virgin olive oil

½ teaspoon sea salt

¾ teaspoon onion powder

¾ teaspoon smoked paprika

1. Preheat the oven to 400°F, and line a baking sheet with parchment paper.

2. Cut the eggplants into ½-inch rounds. Put them in a large bowl and toss with enough oil to coat.

3. Spread the eggplant out on the baking sheet and sprinkle with salt. Roast for 7 minutes. Flip the slices and sprinkle on the onion powder and paprika. Roast for 5 to 8 minutes more. The eggplant is done when they're golden brown and tender when pierced.

SUBS AND SWAPS: Substitute Italian seasonings for the paprika if you want a more Mediterranean flavor.

LOW FODMAP: Omit the onion powder.

PER SERVING Calories: 103; Saturated Fat: 1g; Total Fat: 4g; Protein: 3g; Total Carbs: 17g; Fiber: 7g; Sodium: 242mg

Fajita Peppers and Onions

Prep time: 10 minutes · ***Cook time:*** 30 minutes · ***Serves:*** 4

NUT FREE | VEGAN

Oven-roasted fajitas are a batch cook's best friend! Rich in essential vitamins, minerals, and flavor, they store well in the refrigerator and can quickly be added to many dishes. Breakfast eggs, lunch tacos, or dinner enchiladas—they're already cooked and waiting to be added. To make it a meal, toss atop Chicken Fajitas Bowl (page 105), pair with Huevos Deliciosos con Salsa (page 64) or Herbed Drumsticks (page 104).

5 bell peppers of different colors—red, orange, green, and yellow

1 onion

1 to 2 tablespoons avocado oil or extra-virgin olive oil

½ teaspoon chili powder

½ teaspoon smoked paprika

½ teaspoon onion powder

½ teaspoon garlic powder

½ teaspoon ground cumin

½ teaspoon sea salt

¼ teaspoon cayenne pepper (optional)

1. Preheat the oven to 400°F. Line a baking sheet with parchment paper.
2. Cut the bell peppers and onion into thin strips. In a large bowl, add the peppers and onions, pour in the avocado oil, and toss to coat. In a small bowl, mix the chili powder, paprika, onion and garlic powders, cumin, salt, and cayenne, if using. Sprinkle the spice mix on the veggies and toss again to evenly coat.
3. Place the veggie mix on the baking sheet in a single layer and roast for about 30 minutes, or until the peppers are as tender as you like.

LOW FODMAP: Leave out the onion and the garlic and onion powders.

PER SERVING Calories: 93; Saturated Fat: 1g; Total Fat: 4g; Protein: 2g; Total Carbs: 15g; Fiber: 3g; Sodium: 243mg

Hippie Collard Greens

Prep time: 5 minutes · *Cook time:* 8 minutes · *Serves:* 4

30 MINUTES | LOW FODMAP | NUT FREE | VEGAN

The hippie in this name comes from the sauce blend used by workers at an organic farm where I once worked. It's a simple and delicious way to dress up veggies, including collards. Collard greens are a gem of the cruciferous family, supporting detoxification while adding an abundance of beta-carotene, vitamins K and C, manganese, calcium, iron, and more. If you've never had collards, note that they're a hardier green, so the finished texture will be a little tougher than spinach, but should still be tender. Serve as a side with any dish—the more greens in your endo-body, the better!

2 pounds collard greens, stemmed (about 2 bunches)

2 tablespoons coconut oil (optional)

2 tablespoons coconut aminos

2 tablespoons nutritional yeast

1. Shred the collard greens into small pieces for quicker cooking.

2. You can cook the greens one of three ways: boil, steam, or sauté in coconut oil, each for 5 to 8 minutes or until the collards are tender and bright green.

3. Strain, if needed, and top the collards with the coconut aminos and nutritional yeast.

SUBS AND SWAPS: Kale, collard greens, and broccoli greens are all heartier greens that cook similarly. If you substitute a more delicate leafy green, like chard, beet greens, or spinach, simply cook for about half the time.

PER SERVING Calories: 158; Saturated Fat: 6g; Total Fat: 9g; Protein: 9g; Total Carbs: 18g; Fiber: 10g; Sodium: 48mg

Summer Herbed Carrots

Prep time: 10 minutes · *Cook time:* 20 to 25 minutes · *Serves:* 2

NUT FREE | VEGAN

Carrots are a delicious starch to add to your meals, lower in carbohydrates but still rich in beta-carotene, potassium, manganese, vitamin K, and fiber of course. Get out of your boring carrot rut with roasting to bring out the flavors, and fresh herbs to get your digestive juices fired up. Carrots are so much more than a boring stick. Serve with Golden Hour Fish Pie (page 101) or Offally Good Sausage (page 67).

4 large carrots (bonus if you can find different colors)
Extra-virgin olive oil
½ teaspoon sea salt
2 teaspoons dried basil
1 teaspoon dried thyme
½ teaspoon onion powder
Fresh lemon juice (optional)

1. Preheat the oven to 400°F.

2. Cut the carrots using a food processor slicer attachment. (Or you can use a mandoline or an old-fashioned knife and cutting board.) Just make sure to slice the carrots into similar-size slices.

3. In a large mixing bowl, toss the carrots with oil to coat, then spread the slices out on a baking sheet and sprinkle with the salt, basil, thyme, and onion powder.

4. Roast for 20 to 25 minutes, depending on the size of the slices, until they're golden around the edges and fork-tender. You may need to stir or flip halfway through, depending on your oven, so peek in after 12 minutes to double-check.

5. Add a squirt of lemon juice for brightness if you prefer, and serve.

SUBS AND SWAPS: You can easily cut these into carrot "fries," if you prefer. Roast a little longer, and toss the carrots with onion powder, garlic powder, salt, and paprika.

LOW FODMAP: Omit the onion powder.

PER SERVING Calories: 123; Saturated Fat: 1g; Total Fat: 7g; Protein: 1g; Total Carbs: 15g; Fiber: 4g; Sodium: 568mg

Rainbow Unicorn Carrot and Beet Shreds

Prep time: 5 minutes · *Cook time:* 8 minutes · *Serves:* 2

30 MINUTES | NUT FREE | VEGAN

Shredded veggies make great coleslaw, but they also make a fantastic cooked dish in no time at all—another magically fast way to expedite veggies onto your plate. Shred your favorites, sauté on the stove until tender, add your favorite seasonings, and you have 2 to 3 cups of veggies for any meal. Try shredding the beets and carrots in a food processor—see how easy chopping veggies is this way?

1 to 2 tablespoons extra-virgin olive oil

4 cups shredded, mixed carrots and beets

½ teaspoon sea salt

1 teaspoon garlic powder

1. Heat the olive oil over medium-high heat.
2. Sauté the carrots and beets until tender, for about 8 minutes.
3. Sprinkle with salt and garlic powder.

LOW FODMAP: Substitute Green Herb Oil for garlic powder.

PER SERVING Calories: 147; Saturated Fat: 1g; Total Fat: 7g; Protein: 3g; Total Carbs: 20g; Fiber: 5g; Sodium: 610mg

CULINARY IDEAS
Egg foo fry: Shred celery, zucchini, and red pepper, scramble 2 eggs, and fry into patties with sesame oil
Garden fry: Shred broccoli, green beans, and beets, sauté in extra-virgin olive oil, top with Green Herb Oil (page 140)
Mexican fry: Shred onion (omit for low FODMAP), cabbage, poblano chiles, bell peppers, sauté in avocado oil, and top with sea salt and ground cumin
Greek fry: Shred yellow squash, zucchini, and red onion (omit for low FODMAP), sauté in olive oil, top with sea salt, oregano, and mint
Dessert fry: Shred carrots and sweet potato, sauté in coconut oil until golden, top with cinnamon, raisins, and a dollop of coconut cream

Broccoli Fried "Rice"

Prep time: 10 minutes · *Cook time:* 8 minutes · *Serves:* 4

30 MINUTES | NUT FREE | VEGAN

The cruciferous family of veggies is known to aid the liver in detoxifying, which is why the more on your plate the better. Broccoli is also a nice alternative to cauliflower for the low-FODMAP crowd, and this recipe jazzes up any blandness. What a delicious way to add more veggies to your plate! To make it a meal, serve with Thai Shrimp Scampi (page 98) or Broiled Maple Sesame Salmon (page 95).

2 medium broccoli heads

4 tablespoons sesame oil, divided

½ teaspoon sea salt

1 teaspoon garlic powder

1 teaspoon ginger powder

1 tablespoon blackstrap molasses

3 tablespoons coconut aminos

2 scallions, chopped

1. Make the "rice:" Roughly chop the broccoli and put it into a food processor. Pulse until the broccoli is about the size of rice grains. You may need to push down the sides once or twice to keep everything evenly distributed.

2. Heat 2 tablespoons of sesame oil in a large skillet over medium-high heat, and toss in the broccoli rice, salt, garlic powder, and ginger powder. Sauté for 3 to 4 minutes, until the broccoli starts to brighten. Add the remaining 2 tablespoons of sesame oil, molasses, and coconut aminos, and sauté for another 3 minutes, until the "rice" is fork tender.

3. Quickly remove the "rice" from heat to prevent sogginess. Top with scallions, and season with more coconut aminos and salt.

MAKE IT FAST: Many grocers sell organic, pre-riced veggies in the freezer section these days. Choose your favorite and make it into fried rice.

LOW FODMAP: Omit the garlic powder and use only the green part of the scallions.

PER SERVING Calories: 203; Saturated Fat: 2g; Total Fat: 14g; Protein: 4g; Total Carbs: 17g; Fiber: 4g; Sodium: 299mg

Cinnamon, Cacao, and Cayenne Cauliflower

Prep time: 10 minutes · *Cook time:* 30 minutes · *Serves:* 4

NUT FREE | VEGAN

Another cruciferous vegetable to brighten your meals, cauliflower is not only liver-supportive, but rich in a variety of antioxidants and polyphenols to promote lower inflammation levels. If you're bored with the usual recipes, try this exotic three-C combination: cinnamon plus cacao plus cayenne—a savory blend reminiscent of mole and a fresh flavor for this much-loved veggie staple. Substitute paprika for the cayenne if you prefer less heat.

1 cauliflower head, chopped into florets

3 tablespoons coconut oil, melted

½ teaspoon cinnamon

½ teaspoon cacao powder

½ teaspoon cayenne pepper

½ teaspoon garlic powder

½ teaspoon sea salt

1. Preheat the oven to 400°F.
2. In a large bowl, toss the florets in coconut oil and spread them out on a baking sheet.
3. In a small bowl, mix together the cinnamon, cacao, cayenne, garlic powder, and salt. Sprinkle the spice mix atop the cauliflower.
4. Roast in the oven for about 30 minutes, or until the cauliflower florets are tender and golden brown at the edges.

LEFTOVERS AND EXTRAS: This recipe works really well as leftovers. You can add it cold to salads or packed lunches, reheat it as a side dish, or mix it in with other veggies for a leftover medley. Consider doubling the recipe every time you make it to save you time.

LOW FODMAP: Omit the garlic powder.

PER SERVING Calories: 146; Saturated Fat: 1g; Total Fat: 11g; Protein: 5g; Total Carbs: 12g; Fiber: 6g; Sodium: 297mg

Twice-Crisped Plantain Medallions

Prep time: 10 minutes · ***Cook time:*** 20 minutes · ***Serves:*** 4

30 MINUTES | LOW FODMAP | NUT FREE | VEGAN

Plantains are one of my favorite starches because of their nutrition and flavor, and their ability to make you feel truly sated. In fact, add ½ cup of plantains to any meal and you won't leave hungry, making this starch a fab blood sugar regulator. Cook green plantains if you like them more like a potato, or let them ripen until they're yellow (as I like them) for the sweeter flavors to emerge. Serve with Hanalei Fish Tacos (page 100), Chicken Fajitas Bowl (page 105), or Offally Good Sausage (page 67) for a meal.

2 to 3 tablespoons coconut oil

2 large yellow plantains, peeled and cut into ½-inch medallions

Sea salt

1. In a medium skillet, heat the coconut oil over high heat.

2. Carefully slide the plantains into the oil and fry in batches, turning when the bottoms are golden brown, for 2 to 3 minutes per side. If you like your plantains soft, remove them now. If you want them crispy, continue to cook to your desired texture.

3. Remove the once-fried plantains from pan, place them between two pieces of parchment paper, and press down with a book, pan, tortilla press, or other flat, weighted object.

4. Place the flattened plantain medallions back in the hot oil and fry for another 1 to 2 minutes per side, until crispy.

5. Sprinkle with salt and any spices you like.

PER SERVING Calories: 153; Saturated Fat: 5g; Total Fat: 5g; Protein: 1g; Total Carbs: 29g; Fiber: 2g; Sodium: 121mg

Perfect Stir-Fry

Prep time: 10 minutes · *Cook time:* 10 minutes · *Serves:* 4

30 MINUTES | NUT FREE | VEGAN

A perfect stir-fry is so versatile! Once you know the basics, you'll realize you can substitute in any ingredients you want, and it can be as salty, spicy, Chinese-, Thai-, or Sri Lankan–flavored as you wish. All it takes are the right spices and a solid heap of endo-healing fats and veggies. Paired with the Ohana Hawaiian Stir-Fry Sauce (page 147), this is one of my favorites. Make sure to make it a meal by adding your choice of protein.

4 tablespoons coconut oil

5 scallions, diced

2 lemongrass stalks, root lightly pounded

1 (2-inch) piece fresh ginger, peeled and diced (or ½ teaspoon ginger powder)

1 large red bell pepper, seeded and cut into thin strips

1 large carrot, cut into thin strips

1 small purple cabbage, cut into thin strips

1 bok choy head, chopped

2 tablespoons coconut aminos

½ teaspoon garlic powder

½ teaspoon red pepper flakes

½ teaspoon sea salt

Few dashes fish sauce

1 cup Ohana Hawaiian Stir-Fry Sauce (page 147)

1 cup fresh bean sprouts

Handful fresh basil leaves

1. In a large skillet set over medium-high heat, heat the coconut oil. Sauté the scallions, lemongrass, and ginger for about 1 minute, until fragrant.

2. Add the bell pepper, carrot, cabbage, bok choy, coconut aminos, garlic powder, red pepper flakes, salt, and fish sauce. Sauté for 5 to 7 minutes, until the veggies are tender, but still crisp.

3. Stir in the Ohana Stir-Fry Sauce, then add the bean sprouts and basil. Toss to warm, and serve immediately.

SUBS AND SWAPS: Choose any veggies you want, really. This recipe basically calls for 5 cups of veggies, chopped into similar sizes.

LOW FODMAP: Use only the green part of the scallion and omit the garlic powder.

PER SERVING Calories: 295; Saturated Fat: 12g; Total Fat: 15g; Protein: 8g; Total Carbs: 34g; Fiber: 8g; Sodium: 597mg

Sweet Sesame Mushrooms and Greens

Prep time: 5 minutes · *Cook time:* 10 minutes · *Serves:* 4

30 MINUTES | NUT FREE | VEGETARIAN

Greens are good for you—you know that. They are loaded with essential vitamins and minerals, phytonutrients, antioxidants, fiber, and are pretty easy to find no matter where you live. The problem many of us face is how to eat enough, and that's why simple sautés help. In this recipe, nutrient-dense mushrooms and greens are paired in a simple sweet sesame sauce any green-eating newbie can appreciate. Serve with Egg Drop Soup (page 62) or Golden Hour Fish Pie (page 101) for a meal.

3 to 4 tablespoons sesame oil

4 cups mushrooms, halved

½ teaspoon sea salt, plus more for seasoning

8 cups bok choy, chopped well for fast cooking

2 tablespoons coconut aminos

2 teaspoons raw honey

2 teaspoons sesame seeds

1. In a large pan set over medium-high heat, heat the sesame oil. Add the mushrooms and salt, and cook for about 5 minutes, until the mushrooms are beginning to brown. Add the bok choy and coconut aminos. Continue to cook until the mushrooms are fully browned and the bok choy is wilted, about 5 minutes more.

2. Season with honey, sesame seeds, and salt.

SUBS AND SWAPS: You can use most any greens or veggies here, which is fun when trying new foods from the farmers' market. Be adventurous.

LOW FODMAP: Use oyster mushrooms as nearly all other mushrooms are high FODMAP.

PER SERVING Calories: 180; Saturated Fat: 2g; Total Fat: 15g; Protein: 5g; Total Carbs: 10g; Fiber: 2g; Sodium: 338mg

Spaghetti Squash Noodles

Prep time: 5 minutes · ***Cook time:*** 45 minutes · ***Serves:*** 4

LOW FODMAP | NUT FREE | VEGAN

You don't need any fancy equipment to make these noodles—they're nature-made. Spaghetti squash is rich in beta-carotene, B-complex vitamins, and fiber, but low in starch, meaning it will fill you up with nutrients without spiking your blood sugar, like wheat noodles. If you're a noodle-loving gal, aim to make one of these per week to have on hand for when cravings strike. Top with Cocoa Beef Ragu (page 110), Green Herb Oil (page 140), or Cashew Cheese (page 145). If you like spaghetti squash as is—like me—consider putting a healthy dollop of grass-fed butter with some sea salt on top.

1 large spaghetti squash

Extra-virgin olive oil

½ teaspoon sea salt

1. Preheat the oven to 400°F.

2. Halve the squash lengthwise and remove the seeds and inner pith.

3. Pour oil on each half and rub to coat evenly. Sprinkle the squash halves with salt and place them facedown on a baking sheet. Add ½ cup of water to the pan to help steam the squash.

4. Bake for 35 to 45 minutes. It's done when you can push on the outside of the squash and it caves slightly.

5. Remove the pan from the oven and let cool slightly for easier handling. Carefully scoop out the flesh of the squash and place it in a bowl, using a fork to fluff apart the strands into noodles.

6. Serve immediately, or store in the refrigerator for 3 to 5 days.

SUBS AND SWAPS: Some of us love spaghetti squash as it is, but if you need a flavor infusion, do a twice bake. After baking the squash as above, remove, flip over, and top with your sauce of choice (marinara, pesto, meat sauce) and put back it in the oven for 20 more minutes. This will help bake in the flavors.

PER SERVING Calories: 123; Saturated Fat: 1g; Total Fat: 8g; Protein: 1g; Total Carbs: 14g; Fiber: 0g; Sodium: 268mg

Roasted Squash Soup

Prep time: 5 minutes · *Cook time:* 60 minutes · *Serves:* 4

NUT FREE

No one likes to cut apart a hard winter squash like butternut. To avoid the chore of peeling, cutting, and seeding, roast the squash whole instead. This way you can benefit from the boom of antioxidants, vitamin B, C, and E, and assortment of minerals without breaking a sweat. Blend it with Bone Broth (page 148) and spices, and suddenly you have a fancy bisque.

1 medium butternut squash (about 4 cups cooked flesh)

1 onion, diced

2 teaspoons coconut oil

4 to 6 cups Bone Broth (page 148)

½ teaspoon garlic powder

1 teaspoon dried rosemary

1 teaspoon dried thyme

½ teaspoon sea salt

1. Preheat the oven to 400°F.

2. With a sharp knife, pierce the squash numerous times through the neck and body. Place it on a baking sheet and roast for 45 to 60 minutes, depending on the size of the squash. It's done when the skin has darkened and you can easily slide a knife all the way through the thickest part of the neck. (See how easy that is?)

3. While the squash is roasting, sauté your onion in coconut oil in a small skillet over medium-high heat, until golden, 5 to 8 minutes.

4. Remove the pan from the oven and let it cool until the squash is safe to handle. Cut the squash in half and scoop out the seeds. (Seeds can be discarded or roasted to eat if you like.) Then, scoop out the flesh.

5. Working in batches, put the flesh in a blender with the onion and enough bone broth to cover. Blend until smooth, adding more broth as necessary for your thickness preference.

6. Pour the blended soup into a large serving bowl and stir in the garlic powder, rosemary, thyme, and salt.

PER SERVING Calories: 151; Saturated Fat: 3g; Total Fat: 5g; Protein: 8g; Total Carbs: 21g; Fiber: 4g; Sodium: 349mg

Baked Apples and Onions

Prep time: 10 minutes · *Cook time:* 25 minutes · *Serves:* 4

30 MINUTES | NUT FREE | VEGAN

Apples and onions are both prebiotic foods, meaning they feed your gut microbes. This means if you're on a low-FODMAP diet they won't work for you. But for the rest of you, they'll offer your gut microbiome a feast! Although apples aren't known for their vitamin or mineral content, what they do showcase are dozens of varieties of polyphenols, making them antioxidant royalty. This side dish pairs well with savory meat dishes, like Offally Good Sausage (page 67), Turkey Burgers (page 107), or Slow-Cooked Kalua Pork and Cabbage (page 113). It's higher in carbohydrates, though, so aim to make it a side rather than the focus of your meal.

1 red onion

3 apples

Coconut oil, melted

¼ to ½ teaspoon sea salt

Unsweetened dried cranberries or raisins (optional)

1. Preheat the oven to 400°F. Line a baking sheet with parchment paper.

2. Slice the onion and apples into ¼-inch to ½-inch rounds. You don't have to peel or core the apples, just slice them into rounds and remove the seeds. Easy!

3. Place the apples and onions on the baking sheet, trying not to stack them on top of one another. Lightly coat them with coconut oil and sprinkle with salt.

4. Roast for 20 to 25 minutes, until golden brown.

5. Top with a small sprinkling of dried cranberries or raisins, if you like.

PER SERVING Calories: 127; Saturated Fat: 3g; Total Fat: 4g; Protein: 1g; Total Carbs: 26g; Fiber: 5g; Sodium: 237mg

Hula Mashed Potatoes

Prep time: 10 minutes · *Cook time:* 60 minutes · *Serves:* 6

LOW FODMAP | NUT FREE | VEGAN

Purple sweet potatoes are a Hawaii favorite, and you can now find them in many major grocery stores. They're packed with one and a half times more anthocyanin (one of the rarer antioxidants, found in purple produce) than blueberries, and about half the starch of white potatoes. Roasting the roots helps develop the sweet flavor and retain the tropical color. This dish is delicious, but make sure it's a small side rather than a huge bowl.

Coconut oil

3 large purple sweet potatoes (about 3 pounds)

1 (12-ounce) can full-fat coconut milk

½ teaspoon sea salt

1 teaspoon cinnamon

Pinch nutmeg

Pinch freshly ground black pepper

Toasted pecans (optional)

1. Preheat the oven to 400°F, and set a rack in the lowest position in your oven.

2. Rub coconut oil over the skin to coat the potatoes, and place on baking sheet (no cutting, stabbing, or aluminum foil necessary). Bake for 45 to 60 minutes. They're done when you can easily stick a knife through the widest part. If they look dry while cooking, drizzle on a little extra coconut oil.

3. Using a clean dish towel to protect your hands from heat, carefully slip the skins off and place the potato flesh in a large bowl. Mix in all the remaining ingredients and use a potato masher to mash to your preferred consistency.

LOW FODMAP: Limit your serving to ½ cup.

MAKE IT FAST: If you don't have the time to roast the potatoes, you can peel them, dice into small pieces, place in a saucepan and add the coconut milk and spices. Cover and let simmer for 8 to 10 minutes, until cooked through. Mash to you preferred consistency.

PER SERVING Calories: 333; Saturated Fat: 13g; Total Fat: 14g; Protein: 5g; Total Carbs: 49g; Fiber: 8g; Sodium: 289mg

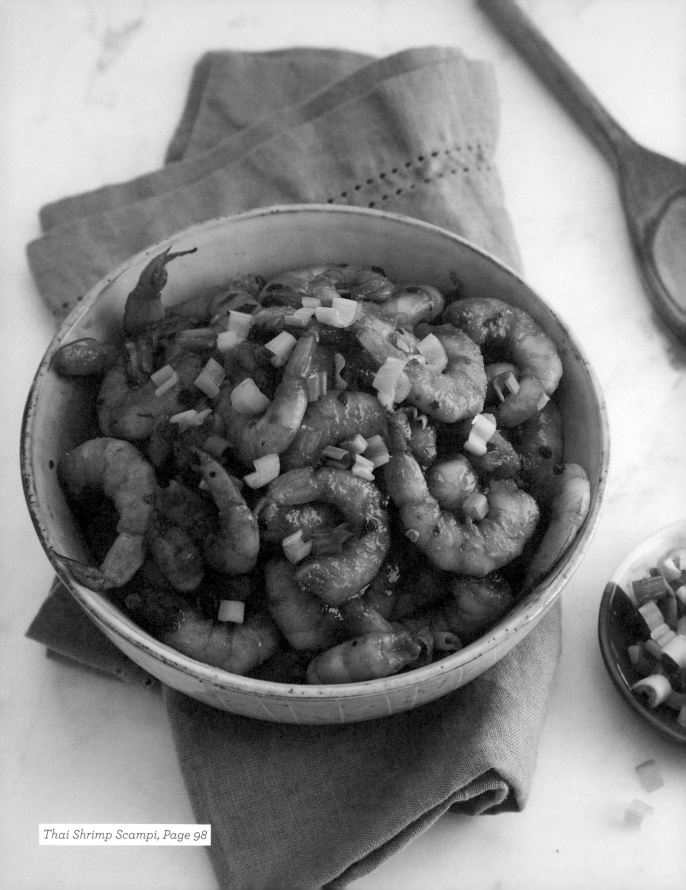

Thai Shrimp Scampi, Page 98

CHAPTER 8

Ocean

I Can't Believe I'm Eating
Sardine Salad

Prep time: 5 minutes · *Serves:* 4

30 MINUTES | NUT FREE

Sardines are delicious, I'm telling you, but a few years ago I may not have thought so, mostly because of their fishy reputation. Truthfully, sardines are similar to tuna, just a tad fishier in flavor and softer in texture. If you're new to sardines you may need a baby step or two in learning to love these best-of-the-best endo foods. Mix them with salmon and herbs and you may not believe how much you love sardines. Already love sardines? Make this salad without any salmon at all—pure sardine goodness!

2 (6-ounce) cans wild-caught salmon, drained

1 (4-ounce) can wild-caught sardines in olive oil, not drained

2 celery stalks, diced

2 scallions, diced

2 tablespoons avocado oil mayonnaise, or Green Herb Oil (page 140)

¼ teaspoon sea salt

1 teaspoon apple cider vinegar

1. Add all the ingredients to a large mixing bowl, including the sardine oil from the can (where remaining omega-3s are hiding out) and stir until well combined.

2. Keeps well in the refrigerator for 2 to 3 days.

LEFTOVERS AND EXTRAS: Serve on a salad, in Nori Wraps (page 94), on plantain chips, celery stalks, or cucumber slices. Add chopped apples, walnuts, and some raisins and turn this into a pseudo-Waldorf salad.

LOW FODMAP: Use only the green part of the scallions.

PER SERVING Calories: 239; Saturated Fat: 4g; Total Fat: 17g; Protein: 22g; Total Carbs: 1g; Fiber: 1g; Sodium: 685mg

Salmon Burgers

Prep time: 5 minutes · *Cook time:* 10 minutes · *Serves:* 2

30 MINUTES | NUT FREE

This salmon recipe is a great stepping stone for any picky eaters out there. Salmon burgers are fried in healthy fat and full of bright flavor that masks the fish for anyone unfamiliar with ocean flavors. Top with Fermented Shreds (page 124) and Fermented Ketchupepper (page 143) sandwiched between two Sun Buns (page 122) and you have yourself a bona-fide Heal Endo—approved salmon burger.

1 (6-ounce) can wild-caught salmon

1 egg

2 tablespoons arrowroot flour

½ red bell pepper, seeded and finely diced

2 scallions, finely diced

¼ teaspoon sea salt

¼ teaspoon garlic powder

1 tablespoon dried parsley

1 tablespoon coconut oil

1. Add the salmon, egg, arrowroot flour, bell pepper, scallions, salt, garlic powder, and parsley to a large mixing bowl and stir until well combined.

2. In a pan over medium-high heat, heat the coconut oil. Quickly form the salmon mixture into patties and place them one by one into the pan, flattening with a spatula.

3. Cook for about 5 minutes per side, flipping when golden brown, pressing again with the spatula, and adding more oil if necessary.

LEFTOVERS AND EXTRAS: These cooked patties keep well in the refrigerator for 3 to 4 days, and are a great ready-made option to add to Nori Wraps (page 94) or as a quick protein to any salad. Double or triple the recipe on Sunday for a week's worth of lunches.

LOW FODMAP: Use only the green part of the scallions, and omit the garlic powder.

PER SERVING Calories: 212; Saturated Fat: 4g; Total Fat: 11g; Protein: 23g; Total Carbs: 5g; Fiber: 1g; Sodium: 573mg

Nori Wraps

Prep time: 15 minutes · *Serves:* 2

30 MINUTES | NUT FREE

Nori Wraps are a great packed lunch for anyone confused about how to live without bread. Nori (pressed sheets of seaweed) is packed with ocean-based minerals and antioxidants, while coldwater fish has those powerful omega-3s I love to talk about. It has protein, fat, nutrients, and is filling and easy to take on the go? Yes, please!

2 (6-ounce) cans wild-caught salmon and/or sardines, or 1 cup seafood leftovers

¼ teaspoon sea salt

2 to 3 tablespoons avocado oil mayonnaise, or Green Herb Oil (page 140)

2 scallions, minced

1 cucumber, julienned

1 red bell pepper, seeded and julienned

¼ cup roughly chopped fresh mint leaves

½ cup diced mango

4 nori sheets

Thai sweet chili sauce (optional)

1. Drain the canned fish and mix it with the salt, mayo, and scallions in a medium bowl.
2. Assemble your wraps by layering the fish, veggies, mint, and mango onto the nori sheets. Top with sweet chili sauce, if using.

MAKE IT FAST: You can easily use leftover seafood of any kind, with lettuce or raw shreds (shredded veggies) and top with your dressing of choice. This is a super simple lunch, and why your favorite veggie shreds are great to keep handy in the refrigerator. Consider carrots, bell peppers, and zucchini.

LOW FODMAP: Use just the green part of the scallions, and use pineapple instead of mango.

PER SERVING Calories: 332; Saturated Fat: 4g; Total Fat: 19g; Protein: 23g; Total Carbs: 17g; Fiber: 5g; Sodium: 572mg

Broiled Maple Sesame Salmon

Prep time: 20 minutes · *Cook time:* 8 to 10 minutes · *Serves:* 2

30 MINUTES | LOW FODMAP | NUT FREE

This flavorful salmon is rich in omega-3s to help quell inflammation. Broiling crisps the nutrient-rich skin while retaining the softness of the interior. Always purchase wild-caught salmon for the correct balance of anti-inflammatory fats. Serve with Broccoli Fried "Rice" (page 81) or Green Bean Frites (page 72) and a salad for a meal.

3 tablespoons sesame oil

3 tablespoons coconut aminos

½ teaspoon sea salt

1 tablespoon pure maple syrup

2 (5-ounce) salmon fillets, skin-on

1. In a small bowl, mix together the sesame oil, coconut aminos, salt, and maple syrup.

2. Put the salmon in a shallow dish and cover with the marinade. Let sit for at least 15 minutes in the refrigerator, but the longer the better.

3. Preheat the broiler when you're ready to cook, and place the rack about 6 inches from the heat.

4. When the broiler is hot, put the salmon in a roasting pan, skin-side down.

5. Broil for 4 minutes, then flip. Brush the remaining marinade on the skin, and broil until the skin is crisp, 4 to 6 minutes more.

LEFTOVERS AND EXTRAS: There's no such thing as too much salmon for the endo-woman. Salmon is easy to make ahead and save for 3 to 4 days in the refrigerator for leftovers. Consider doubling or tripling this recipe.

PER SERVING Calories: 365; Saturated Fat: 3g; Total Fat: 23g; Protein: 29g; Total Carbs: 11g; Fiber: 0g; Sodium: 705mg

Creamy Baked Salmon

Prep time: 10 minutes · *Cook time:* 15 minutes · *Serves:* 4

30 MINUTES | LOW FODMAP | NUT FREE

This rich salmon dish will fill you up for hours with proteins, essential fatty acids, B vitamins, choline, minerals, and more. The rich coconut cream herb sauce blends during baking to create a perfectly decadent dish. Serve over Spaghetti Squash Noodles (page 86) or with a Chopped Green Salad (page 117).

1 pound skinless salmon fillets

1 cup canned heavy coconut cream

½ teaspoon sea salt

½ teaspoon pepper

2 tablespoons chopped fresh dill

2 tablespoons chopped fresh parsley

1. Preheat the oven to 400°F.
2. Place the salmon in a baking dish (the smaller the better, so that the cream is contained around the salmon). Pour the heavy coconut cream over the salmon, and top with the salt, pepper, dill, and parsley.
3. Bake for about 15 minutes, until the cream thickens and the salmon flakes easily. Be careful to not overcook.

SUBS AND SWAPS: If you only have dried herbs, use half the amount listed.

PER SERVING Calories: 466; Saturated Fat: 16g; Total Fat: 24g; Protein: 23g; Total Carbs: 41g; Fiber: 1g; Sodium: 450mg

Easy Scallops

Prep time: 5 minutes · *Cook time:* 10 minutes · *Serves:* 2 or 3

30 MINUTES | NUT FREE

Scallops are like the butter of the sea, and just as rich in nutrients. This makes them great to incorporate into your diet, because who doesn't want healthy, delicious food? Keep the recipe simple to highlight the flavors, and make sure to serve them with plenty of veggies. Scallops significantly reduce in size when cooked; if you're hungry for scallops, or serving very scallop-loving people, consider doubling the recipe, and always serve alongside some veggie sides.

1 pound sea scallops

½ teaspoon sea salt

Freshly ground black pepper

3 tablespoons extra-virgin olive oil

1 garlic clove, grated

1. Blot the scallops dry before cooking (this is the trick to searing the outside). Sprinkle with the salt and pepper.

2. Heal the oil in a large pan over high heat. Add the scallops and cook about 3 minutes, until golden. As you turn the scallops over, add the garlic to the pan as well (and more oil if need). Cook for 2 to 3 minutes more, until both sides are golden and the garlic is fragrant.

3. Serve with extra olive oil and garlic spooned over the scallops.

LOW FODMAP: Omit the garlic.

PER SERVING Calories: 314; Saturated Fat: 3g; Total Fat: 23g; Protein: 25g; Total Carbs: 4g; Fiber: 0g; Sodium: 710mg

Thai Shrimp Scampi

Prep time: 5 minutes · *Cook time:* 10 minutes · *Serves:* 3

30 MINUTES | NUT FREE

A little-known fact about shellfish is how nutrient-dense it is. Four ounces of shrimp offers the full recommended daily allowance of selenium, most of our B12, and lots of choline, copper, and iodine—three nutrients we're often deficient in. Remember to look for sustainably caught or raised options to mitigate chemicals, antibiotic residue, and overfishing. Add these shrimp to Perfect Stir-Fry (page 84) or Sweet Sesame Mushrooms and Greens (page 85) for a meal.

3 tablespoons coconut oil

1 pound shrimp, peeled

½ teaspoon sea salt

½ teaspoon ginger powder

½ teaspoon garlic powder

2 tablespoons Thai sweet chili sauce

2 tablespoons coconut aminos

2 scallions, diced

½ teaspoon red pepper flakes (optional)

1. Heat the coconut oil in a large pan over high heat while you pat dry the shrimp.

2. When the oil is hot, add the shrimp to the pan, sprinkle with the salt, and sauté for 2 to 3 minutes, until the shrimp is just turning pink. Add the ginger and garlic powders, chili sauce, and coconut aminos and cook for 3 to 4 minutes more, until the shrimp are cooked through.

3. Remove the shrimp to a plate with a slotted spoon, and continue to reduce the liquid until it thickens a bit more. Pour the liquid over the cooked shrimp, and top with scallions and red pepper flakes, if using.

LEFTOVERS AND EXTRAS: The cooked shrimp keep in the refrigerator for 3 to 4 days.

LOW FODMAP: Omit the garlic powder and use only the green parts of the scallions.

PER SERVING Calories: 297; Saturated Fat: 12g; Total Fat: 15g; Protein: 32g; Total Carbs: 8g; Fiber: 0g; Sodium: 637mg

Lemon Walnut Mackerel

Prep time: 10 minutes · *Cook time:* 10 to 12 minutes · *Serves:* 4

LOW FODMAP

Mackerel is an omega-rich fish that's a fabulous addition to your anti-inflammatory lifestyle. Full of healthy fats, vitamin D, and selenium, incorporating mackerel into your weekly diet will boost your recovery. Dressed with lemon, walnuts, and avocado oil, this is a healing boost to the system. Serve with Speedy Salad (page 116) or Hippie Collard Greens (page 78).

1 pound mackerel fillets, skin-on

1 tablespoon extra-virgin olive oil

½ cup fresh parsley leaves

3 teaspoons lemon zest

¼ teaspoon sea salt, plus more for seasoning

¼ cup almond flour

½ cup walnuts

4 tablespoons avocado oil

1. Preheat the oven to broil.
2. Place the mackerel in a baking dish, skin-side down, and drizzle with olive oil and season with salt. Broil for 6 to 8 minutes, until the fish is opaque in the center.
3. While broiling, combine the parsley, lemon zest, salt, flour, and walnuts in a food processor, and pulse until the mixture is crumbly. Pour the mixture into a medium bowl and stir in the avocado oil.
4. Evenly spread a layer of the lemon-walnut paste on the tops of the halibut fillets, and return the pan to the oven. Broil for about 4 minutes more, until the crust topping is golden brown.

POWER BOOST: Avoid king mackerel, which may be high in pollutants.

PER SERVING Calories: 513; Saturated Fat: 7g; Total Fat: 45g; Protein: 24g; Total Carbs: 4g; Fiber: 2g; Sodium: 196mg

Hanalei Fish Tacos

Prep time: 30 minutes · ***Cook time:*** 10 minutes · ***Serves:*** 4 to 6

NUT FREE

There's nothing more amazing than watching the sunset over Hanalei Bay while eating fresh-caught fish with friends. Want to recreate this experience? Invite friends over, make this recipe, and enjoy eating this meal together. Community is as healing as food, and that's why it's important to remember that friends belong next to your plate as much as your fork.

3 tablespoons coconut aminos

2 tablespoons fresh lime juice

1 tablespoon fresh grated ginger (from about a 2-inch piece)

½ teaspoon sea salt

2 scallions, thinly sliced

1½ pounds mahi-mahi or other white, flaky fish

1 tablespoon coconut oil

1 romaine lettuce head

1 red bell pepper, seeded and julienned

½ purple cabbage head, shredded

1 cup mango, diced

Coconut Sour Cream (page 144) (optional)

Hot sauce (optional)

1. In a small bowl, mix the coconut aminos, lime juice, ginger, salt, and scallions. Place the fish in a shallow dish and pour over the marinade. Marinate for at least 30 to 60 minutes before cooking.

2. If you have a grill, grill! If you don't, use your stovetop. Heat the coconut oil in a pan over medium-high heat. Remove the fish from the marinade, and fry for 3 to 5 minutes on each side, until the fish is opaque and flakes easily with a fork.

3. Chop the fish into bite-size pieces. Make tacos using romaine leaves as tortillas. Top with the bell pepper, cabbage, mango, and sour cream and hot sauce, if using.

MAKE IT FAST: Use leftover Fajita Peppers and Onions (page 77) to top fish tacos, so you only need to cook the fish and heat the toppings.

LOW FODMAP: Use only the green part of the scallions and swap pineapple for the mango.

PER SERVING Calories: 290; Saturated Fat: 1g; Total Fat: 5g; Protein: 43g; Total Carbs: 19g; Fiber: 4g; Sodium: 370mg

Golden Hour Fish Pie

Prep time: 10 minutes · *Cook time:* 40 minutes · *Serves:* 4

NUT FREE

This low-carb and gluten- and dairy-free version of fish pie is both colorful and satisfying. Cauliflower lends nutrients while thickening the sauce, carrots are a great stand-in for starchy potatoes, and herbs lend flavor and phytonutrients. Cod itself is a great source of easy-to-digest protein, phosphorous, and B vitamins.

3 tablespoons extra-virgin olive oil

1 onion, diced

2 leeks, diced

2 celery stalks, diced

1 pound skinless cod fillets

1 (12-ounce) can full-fat coconut milk, divided

3 bay leaves

1 teaspoon sea salt, divided plus more for seasoning

½ teaspoon black pepper, plus more for seasoning

1 teaspoon garlic powder

1 cauliflower, chopped into florets

1½ tablespoons dried parsley

1½ tablespoons dried tarragon

4 large carrots, boiled until soft

1. Preheat the oven to 400°F.

2. In a large pan over medium-high heat, heat the oil. Add the onion, leeks, and celery to the pan. Sauté for 5 minutes, until they begin to brown, then add the cod, 1 cup of the coconut milk, bay leaves, ½ teaspoon salt, pepper, and garlic powder. Turn the heat to medium and poach the cod until just cooked through. Using a slotted spoon, scoop the fish and veggies from the pan and place on a baking dish, so just the coconut milk broth remains in the pan.

3. Add the cauliflower florets to the hot pan and simmer over medium heat, about 5 minutes, until soft.

4. Using a blender, purée the cauliflower and broth together with the parsley and tarragon to create a thick green sauce. Pour the sauce over the fish in the baking dish.

5. Separately, in a large bowl, mash the cooked carrots with the remaining ½ teaspoon of salt and any left in the can of coconut milk, to your preferred consistency, seasoning with more salt and pepper as desired.

6. Spread the carrot mash over the top of the fish in the baking dish, and bake for 20 to 25 minutes, until the top starts to brown.

LOW FODMAP: Use parsnips instead of cauliflower, red bell pepper in place of the onion, omit the garlic powder, and use only the green parts of the leek leaves rather than the white bulb.

PER SERVING Calories: 486; Saturated Fat: 20g; Total Fat: 32g; Protein: 27g; Total Carbs: 30g; Fiber: 9g; Sodium: 672mg

Chicken Fajitas Bowl, Page 105

CHAPTER 9

Land

Herbed Drumsticks

Prep time: 5 minutes · **Cook time:** 25 to 30 minutes · **Serves:** 2 or 3

30 MINUTES | NUT FREE

Drumsticks are always a crowd pleaser. Coated in phytonutrient-rich herbs, they're mellow, easy to digest, and are rich in glycine from the skin and bone. Serve with any of your favorite plant recipes from this book. Unless you're buying truly free-range birds (which are very pricey), I recommend limiting how much poultry you eat because of the high omega-6 content, making this an inflammation-provoking meat. If you really love chicken (or turkey) and want to eat it often, make sure to balance it out with equal portions of coldwater fatty fish, like salmon, mackerel, or sardines, to contribute extra omega-3s.

1 pound chicken drumsticks, about 4

¼ teaspoon sea salt

½ teaspoon dried basil

½ teaspoon dried thyme

½ teaspoon dried oregano

½ teaspoon onion powder

1. Preheat the oven to 400°F.

2. Place the chicken in a baking dish. Mix together the salt, basil, thyme, oregano, and onion powder. Sprinkle the spice mixture over the chicken to evenly coat.

3. Bake for 25 to 35 minutes, or until cooked through. The juices should be clear, not pink, when the chicken is pierced with a sharp knife.

LEFTOVERS AND EXTRAS: If you have leftovers, you can easily shred them and top a salad or toss in lettuce wraps. This chicken recipe is versatile and mixes well with almost any other flavors.

LOW FODMAP: Omit the onion powder.

PER SERVING Calories: 214; Saturated Fat: 3g; Total Fat: 11g; Protein: 24g; Total Carbs: 1g; Fiber: 0g; Sodium: 670mg

Chicken Fajitas Bowl

Prep time: 10 minutes · *Cook time:* 45 minutes · *Serves:* 4

NUT FREE

This is a recipe to practice your newly acquired batch cooking skills. You'll have food prepped and ready, so you can throw together this meal in no time at all. Bone-in meats offer important amino acids such as glycine (similar to bone broth) to support muscle and joint healing, as well as detoxification. Pair this with a side salad.

4 chicken thighs, bone-in

½ teaspoon sea salt

½ teaspoon garlic powder

1 teaspoon smoked paprika

1 teaspoon dried oregano

Fajita Peppers and Onions (page 77)

1 avocado, sliced

Coconut Sour Cream (page 144) (optional)

Scallions, chopped (optional)

Salsa (optional)

1. Preheat the oven to 400°F.

2. Place chicken thighs in a baking dish, sprinkle with the salt, garlic powder, paprika, and oregano, and bake for 35 to 45 minutes or until cooked through (the juice should be clear, not pink, when poked with a sharp knife).

3. Prepare the Fajita Peppers and Onions and add them to the oven when the chicken has about 30 minutes more to cook.

4. To serve, pair the fajita veggies with a chicken thigh, either shredded or whole, and round out with avocado slices and coconut sour cream, scallions, and salsa, if using.

MAKE IT FAST: To really make this meal fast, batch cook the chicken and the Fajita Peppers and Onions ahead of time. If you make everything on the weekend, you'll have 2 to 3 dinners ready to go with a simple reheat, rather than a big evening dinner cook.

LOW FODMAP: Omit the garlic powder and the white parts of the scallions. Also, leave out the onions from the Fajita Peppers and Onions.

PER SERVING Calories: 403; Saturated Fat: 7g; Total Fat: 28g; Protein: 23g; Total Carbs: 20g; Fiber: 8g; Sodium: 543mg

Thai Coconut Chicken Soup

Prep time: 10 minutes · *Cook time:* 25 minutes · *Serves:* 4

30 MINUTES | NUT FREE

Bone broth is the ingredient that sets an average soup apart from an excellent soup. Its richness and complex variety of minerals turn soup into a nutrient bomb. Thai spices such as kaffir lime leaf, lemongrass, ginger, and turmeric are additional anti-inflammatory aids. I like to add more veggies than traditional soups (are you surprised?) to make it a meal. Kaffir lime leaves have become more readily available in supermarkets and health food stores, plus you can also buy them online.

1 tablespoon coconut oil

1 onion, chopped

2 lemongrass stalks, root lightly pounded, cut into 2-inch pieces

1 (2-inch) piece fresh ginger, chopped

1 (2-inch) piece fresh turmeric root, chopped, or ½ teaspoon dried turmeric

4 boneless chicken thighs, cut into strips

2 cups mushrooms, chopped

2 cups bell peppers, any colors, seeded and chopped

2 cups zucchini, chopped

6 cups Bone Broth (page 148)

1 (12-ounce) can full-fat coconut milk

4 kaffir lime leaves or 3 teaspoons lime zest

1 tablespoon fresh lime juice

1 tablespoon fish sauce

4 tablespoons coconut aminos

1 teaspoon sea salt

1. In a large pot over medium-high heat, add the onion, lemongrass, ginger, and turmeric and sauté for about 5 minutes.

2. Add the chicken thighs, mushrooms, bell peppers, and zucchini to the pot, and sauté until the chicken is nearly cooked, about 3 to 5 minutes.

3. Add the bone broth, coconut milk, lime leaves, lime juice, fish sauce, coconut aminos and salt. Simmer, covered, for 10 to 20 minutes so the flavors blend.

MAKE IT FASTER: Soups like this are quick and easy if you have bone broth on hand, which is why I recommend having extra bone broth in the freezer to make life easier.

LOW FODMAP: Leave out the onion and mushrooms.

PER SERVING Calories: 596; Saturated Fat: 28g; Total Fat: 45g; Protein: 30g; Total Carbs: 20g; Fiber: 4g; Sodium: 909mg

Turkey Burgers with Cashew Cheese

Prep time: 10 minutes · *Cook time:* 16 minutes · *Serves:* 4

30 MINUTES | NUT FREE

One way to get reluctant veggie-eaters to have more is to…well…hide them. And what better place than inside a beloved burger? Mixed with garden herbs, these burgers are far from boring. Top with Cashew Cheese (page 145), enjoy it alongside your favorite salad, and you'll think you're at a trendy LA cafe. If you have time, refrigerate the meat mixture for at least one hour after step 1 to allow the flavors to blend. You can even make the mixture a day ahead.

½ **small red onion**

1 **garlic clove**

1 **red bell pepper, seeded and roughly chopped**

1 **pound ground turkey thighs**

½ **teaspoon sea salt**

1 **teaspoon dried thyme**

1 **teaspoon dried sage**

2 **cups spinach**

1 **small handful fresh basil leaves, or**
   1 **tablespoon dried**

1 **tablespoon coconut oil**

1 **romaine lettuce head for wraps**

Cashew Cheese (page 145)

1. Process the onion, garlic, and bell pepper in a food processor until fine. Add the ground turkey, salt, thyme, sage, spinach, and basil, and process again until everything is well combined.

2. In a large skillet over medium-high heat, heat the coconut oil. Form the meat mixture into 4 patties and cook for 7 to 8 minutes per side, until browned.

3. Place each cooked burger on a romaine lettuce leaf "wrap" and top with Cashew Cheese (page 145), if using.

SUBS AND SWAPS: You can use any ground meat you prefer. 100 percent grass-fed beef or lamb, for example, are often much easier to find (and more affordable) than 100 percent pastured turkey, which can be very expensive.

PER SERVING Calories: 314; Saturated Fat: 7g; Total Fat: 19g; Protein: 25g; Total Carbs: 13g; Fiber: 3g; Sodium: 386mg

Meatloaf Muffins with Apples and Beets

Prep time: 5 minutes · *Cook time:* 20 minutes · *Serves:* 4 to 6

NUT FREE

Meatloaf sounds so old-fashioned—which is a good thing when we remember that folks in the old days weren't dealing with the proliferation of chronic diseases we new-fangled folk face. Truthfully, before canned foods and microwave dinners, our grandparents ate well: Solid meals of meat, veggies, and fats, no snacking, and enjoying one another's company at the dinner table. This is my revamped meatloaf, with added veggies for flavor and nutrients. You add the music from the radio.

Coconut oil, for greasing
1 medium beet
1 medium apple
1½ pounds ground beef
1 teaspoon sea salt
1 teaspoon onion powder
½ teaspoon garlic powder
1 tablespoon dried thyme
1 tablespoon gluten-free Worcestershire sauce

1. Preheat the oven to 400°F. Grease a 12-cup muffin tin with coconut oil.

2. Roughly chop the beet and apple, add them to your food processor, and process until the fruit is thoroughly mashed. Add the ground beef, salt, onion and garlic powders, thyme, and Worcestershire sauce to the food processor, and pulse until combined, stopping as needed to scrape down the sides.

3. Spoon the mixture into the muffin cups and bake for about 20 minutes, or until cooked through. The muffins will be bright pink, so if you're unsure if they are done, poke one with a fork through the center; the juices should run clear.

LEFTOVERS AND EXTRAS: This is a versatile protein dish that goes with almost everything in this book, so having extra on hand will be helpful if you're ever stuck in a hungry jam. They're so simple to make, you can triple the recipe and freeze leftovers to take out as needed for the month.

SUBS AND SWAPS: Swap cauliflower, spinach, or cabbage for the apples and beets for a low-carb option.

LOW FODMAP: Leave out the garlic and onion powders, and use parsnips instead of apples.

PER SERVING Calories: 295; Saturated Fat: 6g; Total Fat: 13g; Protein: 33g; Total Carbs: 12g; Fiber: 2g; Sodium: 604mg

Goji Beef Chili

Prep time: 10 minutes · *Cook time:* 35 minutes · *Serves:* 6

NUT FREE

Beanless chili is a staple in our house because it's so easy to throw together, it's rich in amino acids, it has plenty of veggies, it's filling, and there are always leftovers to spare. This recipe is my favorite, complete with smoky chilies and bright bursts of goji berries.

1 to 2 tablespoons extra-virgin olive oil

1 onion, diced

1 pound ground beef or Offally Good Sausage (page 67) mix

2 green bell peppers, seeded and diced

1 large zucchini, diced

1 (28-ounce) jar roasted tomatoes

3 tablespoons tomato paste

4 cups Bone Broth (page 148)

1 (6-ounce) can ancho chilies or chipotle peppers

½ cup goji berries

½ teaspoon sea salt

1 tablespoon chili powder

2 teaspoons cumin

1 teaspoon smoked paprika

1 teaspoon dried oregano

1 teaspoon garlic powder

1. Heat the oil in a pot over medium heat. Add the onion and sauté for 6 to 7 minutes, until lightly golden.

2. Add the meat, bell peppers, and zucchini to the pot, and cook over medium-high heat, crumbling the meat with a wooden spoon, until it is browned, 6 to 8 minutes.

3. Add the tomatoes, tomato paste, bone broth, ancho chilies, goji berries, salt, chili powder, cumin, paprika, oregano, and garlic powder, and bring everything to a simmer. Cover and cook for about 20 minutes for the flavors to develop.

LOW FODMAP: Leave out the garlic powders, and use diced red bell pepper instead of the onion.

PER SERVING Calories: 287; Saturated Fat: 4g; Total Fat: 12g; Protein: 25g; Total Carbs: 24g; Fiber: 5g; Sodium: 549mg

Cocoa Beef Ragu

Prep time: 10 minutes · ***Cook time:*** 30 minutes · ***Serves:*** 4

NUT FREE

Ragu is an Italian meat sauce that is fantastic when made with grass-fed meats, olive oil, tons of vegetables and . . . chocolate? Yes, and I argue it's an essential missing ingredient that adds depth and flavor to many tomato-based dishes. This dish tastes even better when it's had a chance to sit overnight in the refrigerator. Serve over Spaghetti Squash Noodles (page 86) for a delightful spaghetti night replacement.

1 tablespoon extra-virgin olive oil

1 large onion, diced

2 garlic cloves, minced

1 pound ground beef, or Offally Good Sausage (page 67) mix

1 teaspoon sea salt

2 cups mushrooms, chopped

1 zucchini, chopped

1 green bell pepper, seeded and chopped

1 (16-ounce) jar crushed tomatoes

3 tablespoons tomato paste

3 cups Bone Broth (page 148)

2 to 3 tablespoons Italian seasoning

2 tablespoons cacao powder

1. In a pot over medium heat, heat the oil. Add the onion and cook, about 5 minutes, until the onion is translucent. Add the garlic to the pot and cook for 1 minute more, until fragrant.

2. Add the meat and salt to the pot, and cook, breaking up the meat with a wooden spoon, until it's crumbled and browning.

3. Add the mushrooms, zucchini, bell pepper, tomatoes, tomato paste, bone broth, Italian seasoning, and cacao powder to the pot. Cover and bring the liquid to a simmer. Simmer for 20 minutes, until the veggies are cooked through.

SUBS AND SWAPS: I often make this at the end of the week with all the random veggies left in the refrigerator, to save money and reduce food waste. Plus, it tastes a bit different every time I make it.

LOW FODMAP: Leave out the garlic and onion.

PER SERVING Calories: 388; Saturated Fat: 7g; Total Fat: 19g; Protein: 35g; Total Carbs: 27g; Fiber: 9g; Sodium: 809mg

Ragu-Stuffed Bell Peppers

Prep time: 5 minutes · *Cook time:* 20 minutes · *Serves:* 4

30 MINUTES | LOW FODMAP | NUT FREE

We seemingly can't get enough vitamin C to offset our abundantly stressful lives, which is why eating fresh fruits and veggies is so necessary. Bell peppers are rich in vitamin C, which is essential for collagen synthesis, gum health (do your gums bleed when you brush them?), and definitely for adrenal support. Stuff the peppers with filling proteins and take them for lunch on the go! Serve this with Zesty Zucchini (page 75), Roasted Fennel (page 74), or pair it with a side salad.

4 cups Cocoa Beef Ragu (page 110)

4 bell peppers, tops removed like little hats

1. Preheat the oven to 400°F.

2. Reheat the Cocoa Beef Ragu in a microwave or in a pan on the stovetop. Spoon the warm mixture into the bell pepper cups.

3. Place on a baking sheet and bake for 15 to 20 minutes, or until the peppers are tender when poked. Serve hot.

LEFTOVERS AND EXTRAS: Leftovers refrigerate well. These peppers make an excellent packed lunch.

PER SERVING Calories: 418; Saturated Fat: 7g; Total Fat: 19g; Protein: 36g; Total Carbs: 36g; Fiber: 11g; Sodium: 812mg

Lamb Meatballs with Minted Tahini Sauce

Prep time: 10 minutes • *Cook time:* 16 minutes • *Serves:* 3

30 MINUTES | NUT FREE

Lamb is one of the easier 100-percent grass-fed meats to find, and has a rich yet delicate flavor. Like other red meats, lamb is rich in zinc, iron, B vitamins, the perfect balance of amino acids, and, when grass-fed, omega-3 fats. Use the right spices and be amazed at how flavorful lamb can be. Still not a fan of lamb? Use any ground meat you prefer. These meatballs pair perfectly with a nice salad.

For the minted tahini sauce

½ **cup tahini**

½ **cup filtered water**

1 **big handful fresh mint leaves**

½ **lemon, juiced**

For the meatballs

1 **pound ground lamb**

½ **red onion, minced finely in the food processor**

½ **teaspoon sea salt**

½ **teaspoon garlic powder**

½ **teaspoon black pepper**

1 **teaspoon cinnamon**

½ **teaspoon paprika**

1 **tablespoon extra-virgin olive oil**

For the minted tahini sauce

Add the tahini, water, mint, and lemon juice to a blender and combine until smooth. Set aside.

For the meatballs

1. Put the lamb, onion, salt, garlic powder, pepper, cinnamon, and paprika in a large mixing bowl.

2. Heat the oil in a large skillet over medium-high heat. Scoop out 1 tablespoon of the lamb mixture at a time and form into small meatballs. Add the meatballs to the skillet and cook for 7 to 8 minutes, turning from time to time, until well browned all over.

3. When the meatballs are finished, portion them out into plates and drizzle the minted tahini sauce on top.

LEFTOVERS AND EXTRAS: If you want to throw these in the oven instead, bake at 400°F for 20 to 25 minutes. You can make these ahead and reheat as needed. It's very simple!

LOW FODMAP: Leave out the garlic powder and substitute some red bell pepper for the onion.

PER SERVING Calories: 585; Saturated Fat: 15g; Total Fat: 47g; Protein: 29g; Total Carbs: 14g; Fiber: 6g; Sodium: 242mg

Slow-Cooked Kalua Pork and Cabbage

Prep time: 5 minutes · *Cook time:* 8 to 10 hours · *Serves:* 15

LOW FODMAP | NUT FREE

Collagen-rich tough cuts of meat are great for healing, but can be hard to chew. Kahlua pork is a slow-cooked melt-in-your-mouth delight, loaded with zinc, iron, B vitamins, and glycine. This recipe makes a lot of food, so freeze the leftovers. You will need a slow cooker or Instant Pot® (or other electric pressure cooker) for this recipe. Smoked sea salt will help recreate the smoky flavor of true Kalua pork, but if you can't find it, the dish will still be delish.

4 to 5 pounds pork shoulder

1 tablespoon smoked sea salt

1 head green cabbage, roughly chopped

1. Place the pork shoulder in a slow cooker and sprinkle it with the salt. Cover and cook on low for 8 to 10 hours (overnight or while you're at work)—the time depends on your slow cooker. You'll know it's ready when the shoulder can easily be shredded with a fork.

2. Add the cabbage about 15 minutes before the pork is done. Don't worry if you miss the window. Just throw some of the pork juice from the pot into a pan with the cabbage and cook it on the stovetop over medium-high heat for about 10 minutes, or until it's soft, and place it back in with the pork.

3. Remove the pork and cabbage from the liquid and place them into a mixing bowl. Using two forks, shred the pork and cabbage together, adding extra liquid or salt as needed.

MAKE IT FAST: (Relatively) Add 1 cup of water to an Instant Pot® with the pork and salt, and cook on high pressure for 90 minutes. Remove the pork from the pot without draining the liquid. Put the cabbage in the pot. Seal the pot and cook on high for 3 minutes. Depressurize. Remove the cabbage and shred it with the pork as in step 3.

POWER BOOST: Save the liquid from the pork to use as a bone broth substitute in sauces, gravies, or other dishes to add flavor and nutrients. This liquid is high in anti-inflammatory glycine and easy-to-digest amino acids, just like bone broth.

PER SERVING Calories: 382; Saturated Fat: 10g; Total Fat: 29g; Protein: 25g; Total Carbs: 4g; Fiber: 2g; Sodium: 222mg

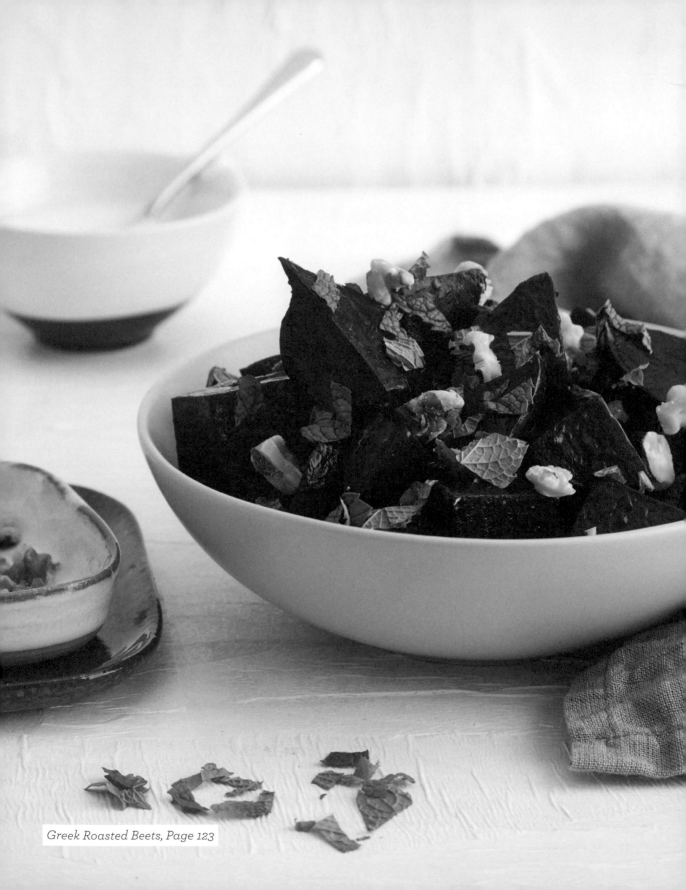

Greek Roasted Beets, Page 123

Salads and Snacks

Speedy Salad

Prep time: 10 minutes · *Serves:* 2

30 MINUTE | VEGAN

To become a salad aficionado you must stop seeing it as "low calorie," and instead as a nutrient-dense and delicious meal option. Dress your salad with nuts and fruit, fill it out with fresh local greens instead of iceberg lettuce, be creative with ingredients and flavors, and always pour on liberal amounts of fat. This is how salads should be. Add any protein you want to make it a meal—think sardine salad, roasted chicken, stuffed peppers, or any other meat dish.

5 cups leafy mix of choice, such as lettuce, kale, arugula, radicchio, or any other leafy greens you love

1 cup fresh shreds of choice, such as carrots, beets, fennel, apple, or zucchini

¼ cup toasted nuts, chopped

2 tablespoons dried fruit or ½ cup fresh fruit

Fertility Goddess Dressing (page 142) or Harvest Moon Raspberry Balsamic Dressing (page 141)

1. Wash and spin or pat dry the greens.
2. Add the shreds—just a fancy way of saying shredded or finely chopped veggies.
3. Add the nuts and fruit, and drizzle with the salad dressing. Speedy and simple!

PER SERVING Calories: 282; Saturated Fat: 2g; Total Fat: 15g; Protein: 8g; Total Carbs: 34g; Fiber: 8g; Sodium: 155mg

CULINARY IDEAS
Herbed: radicchio + arugula + grapefruit + hazelnuts
Hearty: lettuce + kale + pistachios + dried cranberries
Classic: shredded beets + romaine + avocado + raisins
Mediterranean: spring mix + cucumber + figs + mint + toasted almonds

Chopped Green Salad

Prep time: 10 minutes · *Serves:* 2

30 MINUTE | NUT FREE | VEGAN

Chopped salads are hearty and satisfying, and this one packs a nutrient punch. Fresh greens offer a wealth of antioxidants, fresh lemon and greens offer detox support, and fiber feeds you and your gut microbiome. This salad is phytonutrient-rich and liver-supporting. Add chopped bacon, hardboiled eggs, roasted chicken, turkey burgers, or any protein you like to make this a meal. If you tolerate feta or chèvre it might be nice on top, or try some Harvest Moon Raspberry Balsamic Dressing (page 141).

1 small zucchini

1 small cucumber

1 green apple

1 avocado

2 celery stalks

4 tablespoons toasted pistachios

2 tablespoons golden raisins

Sea salt

Fertility Goddess Dressing (page 142)

1. Wash and chop the zucchini, cucumber, apple, avocado, and celery into small pieces. (Hence, chopped salad.) This is a great time to work on your *Top Chef* knife skills! Chop, chop, chop.

2. Toss the chopped fruits and vegetables together in a large bowl with the pistachios, raisins, and salt.

3. Dress with liberal amount of Fertility Goddess Dressing, or your dressing of choice.

LOW FODMAP: Leave out the green apple. Use only ⅛ avocado per serving.

MAKE IT FAST: If you have a food processor, you can pulse the veggies together about 10 times, until they're all roughly chopped and combined.

PER SERVING Calories: 464; Saturated Fat: 5g; Total Fat: 33g; Protein: 8g; Total Carbs: 44g; Fiber: 13g; Sodium: 175mg

Asian Coleslaw Shreds

Prep time: 10 minutes · *Serves:* 4

30 MINUTE | NUT FREE | VEGAN

Coleslaw is hands-down the easiest way to eat more veggies—if you have a food processor. You just push any veggie through and out comes perfectly shredded coleslaw; all you have to do is dress it. This makes it a breeze to get 2 to 3 cups of veggies on your plate quickly. This is my favorite mix, an Asian-inspired coleslaw with the perfect amount of sweet and heat. To make it a meal, add any protein you want. Think salmon cakes, Thai shrimp, honey sesame salmon, or chicken.

1 small purple cabbage head

1 large fennel bulb

2 large carrots

½ cup mango, frozen and defrosted, or fresh

2 tablespoons sesame oil

2 tablespoons coconut aminos

2 tablespoons fresh lime juice

1 teaspoon red pepper flakes

¼ teaspoon sea salt

1. Shred the purple cabbage, fennel, and carrots through your food processor's fine shred attachment. If you don't have a food processor, use a box grater.

2. Dice the mango and toss it together with the shredded veggies in a large bowl.

3. In a small bowl, whisk together the sesame oil, coconut aminos, lime juice, red pepper flakes, and salt.

4. Toss the slaw with the dressing.

LOW FODMAP: Omit the mango.

PER SERVING Calories: 169; Saturated Fat: 1g; Total Fat: 7g; Protein: 4g; Total Carbs: 26g; Fiber: 9g; Sodium: 228mg

CULINARY IDEAS
Classic: red cabbage + green cabbage + carrots + Fertility Goddess Dressing (page 142)
Liver loving: beets + carrots + parsley + lemon juice + olive oil + sea salt
Green machine: zucchini + broccoli + avocado with Fertility Goddess Dressing (page 142)
Garden fresh: cucumber + apple + jicama with Green Herb Oil (page 140)

Nori Crisps

Prep time: 10 minutes · **Cook time:** 30 minutes · **Serves:** 8

LOW FODMAP | VEGAN

Nori is a sea vegetable we should all eat because of its amazing nutrient profile: calcium, copper, iron, magnesium, manganese, phosphorus, potassium, selenium, zinc, vitamins B, C, D, E, and K, plus an abundance of polyphenols! Sadly, it's hard to eat enough when the premade snacks are so pricey (and a plastic packaging nightmare), which is why making your own is such a great idea These are way more satisfying, and just as crispy. Eat them with a dollop of smoked salmon or sardine salad, crumble them into a salad, or use them as a bun replacement.

Sesame oil

16 raw nori sheets (many stores sell packs of 50)

Sea salt

Red pepper flakes (optional)

Sesame seeds (optional)

1. Preheat the oven to 300°F.
2. Pour a dollop of sesame oil on a dinner plate and set aside.
3. Place 1 nori sheet on a cutting board and, using a basting or pastry brush, wet the entire sheet with water.
4. Quickly place another nori sheet on top. Repeat until you have a stack of 4 wet nori sheets. Set aside.
5. Repeat three more times, until all 16 nori sheets have been layered into 4 stacks.
6. Cut each stack into 8 squares, making 32 crisps total.
7. Now, one by one, smear the top of each stack through the sesame oil so it's lightly and evenly coated. Place the sheets oiled-side up on a baking sheet. Sprinkle with salt, red pepper flakes, and sesame seeds, if using.
8. Bake for about 20 minutes, until the stacks are crisp all the way through.

LEFTOVERS AND EXTRAS: Store in sealed jar for 2 to 3 days unrefrigerated, or 1 to 2 weeks in the refrigerator.

PER SERVING Calories: 35; Saturated Fat: 0g; Total Fat: 2g; Protein: 2g; Total Carbs: 2g; Fiber: 2g; Sodium: 41mg

Activated Nuts and Seeds

Prep time: 3 to 12 hours • *Cook time:* 2 to 4 hours • *Serves:* 12

LOW FODMAP | VEGAN

Nuts are a gray area food because you must be careful of sourcing, quality, and preparation to ensure these energy-rich foods are endo-allies and not enemies. The best way to ensure your nuts are easily digestible and nutrient dense is by activating them to reduce phytates and enzyme inhibitors. Nuts contain a lot of omega-6, so eat them in moderation. Remember to think of nuts as condiments, not meals or snacks. Use them to accent a meal instead of eating five handfuls as a meal replacement.

1 cup of nuts or seeds, such as almonds, hazelnuts, macadamias, pecans, walnuts, pine nuts, pumpkin seeds, sunflower seeds, or cashews

Sea salt

3 cups of filtered water

1. Choose any and all of your favorite nuts and seeds. Soak them for 10 to 12 hours in liberally salted water—except cashews, which should soak just 3 to 6 hours, or they will become slimy.

2. Strain and rinse the nuts.

3. If you have a dehydrator, spread the nuts on trays and dehydrate for 12 to 24 hours.

4. If you're using an oven, set it to the lowest possible temperature, spread the nuts and seeds on baking sheets, and bake until the nuts are fully dehydrated, stirring occasionally. This may take 2 to 4 hours, depending on how low your oven temperature goes.

5. It's important the nuts are fully dry and crispy before you remove them from the heat, to reduce spoilage. You'll know they're done when they're crisp as can be without tasting burnt.

6. Let them cool completely. Store in freezer-safe bags or jars in the freezer for you to grab as you need for recipes throughout the month.

LEFTOVERS AND EXTRAS: Activating and dehydrating nuts isn't labor intensive, but it does take some planning, which is why I recommend making a large batch each time. Make this recipe with 1 to 2 pounds of your favorite nuts and seeds and you'll have enough for a month.

POWER BOOST: Toss activated nuts or seeds with truffle oil, salt, and rosemary, and roast at 350°F for 5 minutes.

PER SERVING (¼ CUP) Calories: 174; Saturated Fat: 1g; Total Fat: 15g; Protein: 6g; Total Carbs: 6g; Fiber: 4g; Sodium: 78mg

Sun Buns

Prep time: 10 minutes · *Cook time:* 45 to 60 minutes · *Serves:* 5

VEGAN

I needed to find a bread replacement when I switched to a grain-free diet. It's just so easy to grab a slice of bread, put some protein on it, and toast it when I'm in a rush. Sun Buns were the solution I stumbled upon, so named because of their sunny color. Full of beta-carotene and fiber rich, they keep well in the refrigerator for four to five days.

2 cups cooked sweet potato

½ cup almond flour

½ cup coconut flour

4 tablespoons arrowroot starch

2 tablespoons chia seeds

½ teaspoon sea salt

¼ teaspoon baking powder

¼ teaspoon baking soda

1 tablespoon apple cider vinegar

½ cup nuts or seeds of choice

1. Preheat the oven to 350°F. Line a baking sheet with parchment paper.

2. Place the sweet potato, almond and coconut flours, starch, chia seeds, salt, baking powder and soda, vinegar, and nuts in a food processor and blend them into a sticky dough. If you prefer the nuts or seeds whole, mix them in after the dough is blended; otherwise you can add them to the food processor as well.

3. Shape into 10 little 3-inch buns (they'll look more like cookies) and place them on the baking sheet. Cut a crisscross pattern into the top of each. This is not just for aesthetics, rather it's essential to vent the steam and help them cook evenly in the center, so don't skip this crisscross step.

4. Bake for 45 to 60 minutes, or until the insides are soft but not gooey. After 45 minutes of baking, check for doneness (buns shouldn't be gooey in the middle), and if more time is needed place the buns back in oven for an additional 5 to 10 minutes. If you make the buns bigger, simply cook for longer.

5. Cool to room temperature to fully set. Reheat in the toaster.

LOW FODMAP: For a low-FODMAP diet, the serving size is one bun instead of two.

PER SERVING Calories: 229; Saturated Fat: 2g; Total Fat: 9g; Protein: 7g; Total Carbs: 32g; Fiber: 11g; Sodium: 283mg

Greek Roasted Beets

Prep time: 10 minutes · *Cook time:* 50 minutes · *Serves:* 4
VEGAN

Beets are a veggie that deserve our *love*. They're phytonutrient-rich, available locally almost everywhere, and a terrific boost for your liver. The only problem is they can taste like dirt—literally. Don't give up until you've tried this recipe! Cool, tart coconut sour cream, refreshing fresh mint, and caramelized sweet beets combine for a chilled pink summer salad you're guaranteed to love.

Extra-virgin olive oil

4 large beets, or 8 small

¼ cup chopped fresh mint

½ cup Coconut Sour Cream (page 144), or coconut yogurt

¼ teaspoon sea salt

Fresh mint, roughly chopped

½ cup chopped toasted walnuts

1. Preheat the oven to 400°F.

2. Rub oil on the beets, place them on a baking sheet, drizzle with a little extra oil, and roast them whole in the oven. No peeling, chopping, or covering in aluminum foil needed!

3. Large beets may bake for 40 to 50 minutes, whereas smaller beets require less time. They're done when you can smoothly stick a knife through them.

4. When roasted, remove the beets from oven, let them cool, and put them in the refrigerator to chill.

5. When chilled, cut into cubes and put in a serving bowl. Mix in coconut sour cream or yogurt, sprinkle on salt, and top with fresh mint only when you're ready to serve. Top with toasted walnuts for a fancy addition.

MAKE IT FAST: Cut the beets into 1-inch cubes and roast for about half the time, 25 minutes or so, until tender.

PER SERVING Calories: 236; Saturated Fat: 2g; Total Fat: 14g; Protein: 7g; Total Carbs: 25g; Fiber: 5g; Sodium: 285mg

Fermented Shreds

Prep time: 10 minutes · *Ferment time:* 3 to 10 days · *Makes about 1 quart*

VEGAN

Ferments are so popular, yet it seems to be one of the top foods I see women hesitate to tackle. Why? Probably because fermenting is unfamiliar and can be finicky (like dealing with any living thing), but certainly not because it's hard. Fermenting is actually deceivingly easy, super cheap, and a fun new way to connect with your food—once you get the hang of it. To see for yourself, try this recipe.

1 medium green cabbage, shredded

2 apples, shredded

2 carrots, shredded

2 tablespoons sea salt

1. Wash your hands well so you don't contaminate your ferment.

2. In a large mixing bowl, mix together the shredded cabbage and apples. Add the salt and get ready to flex your hand muscles by massaging the shreds. Squeeze, pack, and knead the mixture for 5 minutes—drawing out the water.

3. Transfer the veggies and all the salty water that's been pulled out (called brine) into a sterilized ½-gallon Mason jar, and use your fist, a large spoon, or a wooden dowel to pack the veggies down, submerging them under the brine.

4. To *keep* them submerged, you'll need to place a weight on them. You can buy fermentation weights, or you can be creative for free. A sterilized rock, glass paperweight, or small glass jar filled with water work well. Put them inside the Mason jar, on top the veggies. If they're still not submerged, mix 1 teaspoon salt into 1 cup water and pour over the top.

5. Cap the jar loosely with the lid, so the contents can breathe, and sit on your counter (out of the sun) for 3 to 10 days. The longer it sits, the more fermented and sour it will be, so feel free to taste it every day until you feel it's ready.

SUBS AND SWAPS: You can ferment any vegetable, literally, so have fun with your adventure! Overall, the basic premise is the same: Pull water out of your veggies, and make sure they're submerged in the brine.

LOW FODMAP: Leave out the apples.

PER SERVING (¼ CUP) Calories: 32; Saturated Fat: 0g; Total Fat: 0g; Protein: 1g; Total Carbs: 8g; Fiber: 2g; Sodium: 718mg

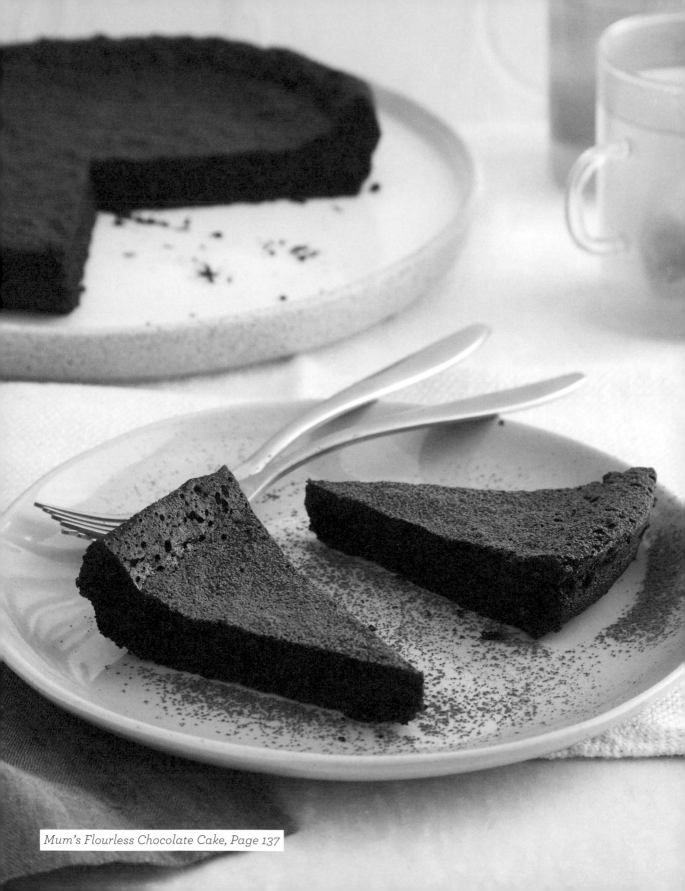

Mum's Flourless Chocolate Cake, Page 137

Drinks and Desserts

Adaptogen Herbal Iced Tea

Prep time: 5 minutes · *Steep time:* overnight · *Makes 4 cups*

LOW FODMAP | NUT FREE | VEGAN

Adaptogens are herbs known for their ability to support the adrenals and the body's stress response system. They nourish and strengthen the adrenals, rather than stimulate them, as caffeine or sugar do. Most of us could definitely use some nourishment, I think. Adaptogens work well over long periods of time, so if you don't notice the effects right away, give it a month and see if you feel more resilience. Schisandra berries come from the Near East and Far East, and have a complex flavor. You can get them at health food stores and online.

2 tablespoons schisandra berries

½ cup hibiscus tea leaves

¼ cup spearmint tea leaves

2 tablespoons holy basil (tulsi) leaves

4 cups boiling water

Pure maple syrup (optional)

1. Place the berries, hibiscus, spearmint, and basil in a saucepan and pour the boiling water over them. Let steep overnight.

2. Strain the tea. Taste and lightly sweeten with maple syrup, if using.

3. Pour the infusion over glasses filled with ice. This tea also keeps well in refrigerator for 3 to 4 days.

MAKE IT FAST: Steeping overnight releases more nutrients, but isn't necessary for you to enjoy this ice tea. Simply steep all the ingredients for 10 to 20 minutes, and pour over ice.

PER SERVING (1 CUP) Calories: 0; Saturated Fat: 0g; Total Fat: 0g; Protein: 0g; Total Carbs: 0g; Fiber: 0g; Sodium: 0mg

Nettle Tea Blood Infusion

Prep time: 10 minutes · *Steep time:* overnight · *Makes 1 quart*

LOW FODMAP | NUT FREE | VEGAN

Nettle tea is incredibly nutrient dense, with plenty of iron, B vitamins, K1, flavonoids, and more. Red raspberry leaf is also quite mineral-rich, and may help support estrogen metabolism. And although the molasses contains sugar, it's worth it (unless you have severe blood sugar issues) due to the extra iron, potassium, magnesium, and other minerals. One quart of this tea may contain upwards of 10mg of iron (the RDA for women is 17mg), and is a precious resource if you suffer from chronic fatigue.

½ cup dried nettles

½ cup dried red raspberry leaf

4 cups boiling water

2 tablespoons blackstrap molasses

1. Place the herbs in a saucepan and pour the boiling water over them. Let the tea steep overnight to really draw out the minerals.

2. In the morning, strain the tea and add the molasses. Enjoy hot or cold.

POWER BOOST: Consider drinking this infusion in the afternoon if you get a midday slump. If you like this tea and feel its benefits, feel free to drink 4 cups every day.

PER SERVING (1 CUP) Calories: 29; Saturated Fat: 0g; Total Fat: 0g; Protein: 0g; Total Carbs: 8g; Fiber: 0g; Sodium: 4mg

Garden Herb Infusion

Prep time: 10 minutes · *Steep time:* 10 minutes · *Serves:* 2

30 MINUTES | LOW FODMAP | NUT FREE | VEGAN

Garden herbs are some of the richest sources of polyphenols we know of, but sometimes it's hard to stretch our creativity to get enough of these anti-inflammatory antioxidants into our daily routine. Instead of reaching for a plastic supplement bottle, try reaching for your garden gloves instead. Growing herbs is easy; it needs nothing more than a sunny window and some water, and yields an excellent polyphenol-rich brew. No garden? Simply stock up at the store. Feel free to replace as much of your daily water with this antioxidant-rich tea as you desire.

1 handful fresh culinary herbs, such as peppermint, oregano, sage, rosemary, thyme, basil, lemon verbena, parsley, or marjoram

3 cups boiling water

1. Place the herbs in a saucepan. Pour the water over the herbs and let it steep 5 to 10 minutes, to your desired flavor profile.

2. Drink every day, hot or cold.

POWER BOOST: In communities around the world that are studied because so many people live healthily and vibrantly into their 100s, people drink herbal teas like this. In Sardinia, they will clip herbs from the garden or wild ones growing on the surrounding hillsides to make a nice afternoon brew.

PER SERVING (1 CUP) Calories: 0; Saturated Fat: 0g; Total Fat: 0g; Protein: 0g; Total Carbs: 0g; Fiber: 0g; Sodium: 0mg

Nut Mylk Any Way

Prep time: 12 hours · *Makes 3 to 4*
VEGAN

Homemade nut mylk is a bit more demanding than storebought, but the effort is worth it for the slew of nutrients, healthy fats, and antioxidants the mylk offers. Not to mention, you avoid the chemical fillers commonly found in boxed options. If you use nut mylks regularly, simply making a routine of soaking and blending nuts every few days (set a reminder if needed) will enable you to seamlessly fold making this beverage into your life. If you're aiming to replace cream in your beverages, make this mylk richer by reducing the amount of water to 2 cups water per 1 cup of soaked nuts.

1 cup nuts or seeds

3 to 4 cups filtered water (depending on how rich you like your mylk)

2 pinches sea salt

Pure maple syrup, blackstrap molasses, or honey (optional)

1. Soak the nuts or seeds, plus a pinch salt, overnight in enough water to cover. Drain and discard the soaking water.

2. Add the nuts, filtered water, another pinch of salt, and sweetener, if using, to a high-powered blender. Blend on high for 1 to 2 minutes, until the nuts are completely "mylked."

3. Strain the liquid through a cheesecloth or fine mesh strainer, and really squeeze the leftover pulp to get all the creaminess out. Sweeten the mylk naturally with the syrup, molasses, or honey, if you like.

4. The mylk will keep in the refrigerator in a glass jar for 2 to 3 days.

LOW FODMAP: Use Brazil nuts, macadamias, pecans, or tiger nuts.

MAKE IT FAST: It's not exactly the same, but if you need nut mylk on the fly blend, 3 tablespoons of any nut butter with 2 cups of filtered water and quickly strain through a cheesecloth.

PER SERVING (1 CUP) Calories: 40; Saturated Fat: 0g; Total Fat: 3g; Protein: 1g; Total Carbs: 0g; Fiber: 0g; Sodium: 86mg

Mocktail Aperitif

Prep time: 5 minutes · *Serves:* 2

30 MINUTES | LOW FODMAP | NUT FREE | VEGAN

In Europe, aperitifs are served before dinner to start your digestive juices flowing . . . and to have time for nice predinner conversation, too. Although we won't be using any alcohol, you can still enjoy the benefits of a premeal sipper to signal your digestive organs to fire up the system. This drink is best served in cute, small glasses, slowly sipped with friends just before eating. Keep the serving size small so you don't overload your tummy with liquid before eating a meal. It should also be pleasantly tart to help you salivate.

1 cup ice

1 lime, juiced

½ ruby red grapefruit, juiced

1 cup sparkling water

1 (2-inch) piece fresh ginger, finely grated

10 dashes herbal bitters (I love Urban Moonshine)

1. Divide the ice and lime and grapefruit juices between 2 glasses.

2. Top each glass with sparkling water, the ginger, and a few dashes of herbal bitters. Stir and serve.

3. If you like the herbal flavor of bitters, feel free to add as much as you'd like to your glass.

PER SERVING Calories: 18; Saturated Fat: 0g; Total Fat: 0g; Protein: 0g; Total Carbs: 5g; Fiber: 0g; Sodium: 2mg

Chilled Berry Parfait

Prep time: 10 minutes · *Serves:* 2

30 MINUTES | LOW FODMAP | VEGAN

Berries are one of the richest sources of antioxidants per gram, so it makes sense to fold them into a fluffy coconut whipped cream and surround them with polyphenol-rich nuts, right? I believe decadence is key with desserts to truly satisfy your craving, without feeling as if you need to binge.

1 (12-ounce) can coconut milk, chilled

1 teaspoon pure vanilla extract

1 teaspoon pure maple syrup

Pinch sea salt

2 cups berries, fresh or frozen and defrosted

4 tablespoons toasted pecans, preferably activated (page 120)

1. Without shaking, remove the can of chilled coconut milk from the refrigerator, open, and scoop out the cream that has risen to the top. Place in a large chilled mixing bowl.

2. Add the vanilla, maple syrup, and salt. Whip the cream with a handheld blender until stiff peaks form, just like whipped cream.

3. In separate bowls, layer the berries, coconut cream, and pecans.

POWER BOOST: Grate some fresh ginger and turmeric on top for an exotic flavor and extra anti-inflammatory and antioxidant properties.

PER SERVING Calories: 532; Saturated Fat: 36g; Total Fat: 50g; Protein: 7g; Total Carbs: 25g; Fiber: 7g; Sodium: 144mg

Chocolate Ganache Pudding

Prep time: 5 minutes · *Chill Time:* 30 to 60 minutes · *Serves:* 4

NUT FREE | VEGAN

Chocolate is rich in polyphenols, avocado in vitamin E, coconut cream in monolaurin for immune system support—all three combine to make one exceptional chocolate pudding. Make a big batch in advance if you know you're going to need a healthy chocolate fix while you transition away from a sweet lifestyle.

2 ripe avocados

2 tablespoons pure maple syrup

⅓ cup raw cacao powder

½ cup heavy coconut cream

½ teaspoon pure vanilla extract

1. Scoop out the fruit of the avocados and add it, the maple syrup, cacao powder, coconut cream, and vanilla to a food processor or blender. Blend until smooth and taste to adjust the sweetness (or cacao content, if you're like me and love chocolate).

2. Pour into a glass container and chill the pudding in the refrigerator for 30 minutes to 1 hour before serving.

LOW FODMAP: You can enjoy 2 tablespoons of this recipe as-is, or you can omit the avocados and substitute 1 cup of heavy coconut cream (rather than just ½ cup). Blend with the rest of the ingredients, and chill for 1 to 2 hours until firm.

PER SERVING Calories: 314; Saturated Fat: 8g; Total Fat: 20g; Protein: 3g; Total Carbs: 35g; Fiber: 6g; Sodium: 80mg

Cacao Butter Bark

Prep time: 10 minutes · *Cook time:* 5 minutes · *Chill time:* 1 hour · *Serves:* 4

30 MINUTES | LOW FODMAP | NUT FREE | VEGAN

Raw cacao butter is the unprocessed sister of cocoa butter, meaning it retains more of its healthy fats, antioxidants, and polyphenols because it hasn't been processed at high heats. It's delightfully rich in all those anti-inflammatory goodies, and makes a decadent vanilla-based desert, especially when paired with bright berries and crunchy seeds.

1 cup raw cacao butter, either chips or chunks

2 tablespoons pure maple syrup

1 teaspoon pure vanilla extract

½ teaspoon sea salt

3 to 4 tablespoons cacao powder (optional), if you prefer chocolate with your butter

2 tablespoons toasted shelled pumpkin seeds

2 tablespoons dried cherries, raisins, or blueberries

1. Heat some water in a pot over the stove on medium heat. When the water begins to simmer, set a heatproof bowl on top of the pot and add the cacao butter to the bowl. Stir as the cacao butter melts and remove from the heat as soon as it's smooth. Transfer the butter to a large mixing bowl.

2. Stir in the maple syrup, vanilla, salt, and cacao powder, if using. Whisk until smooth.

3. Line a baking sheet with parchment paper (including the edges to prevent spillover), and pour in mixture. Using the back of a spoon or a spatula, spread the mixture in the pan to create a thin layer of bark. Sprinkle the top of the bark with seeds and dried fruit, and refrigerate for at least 1 hour, to solidify.

4. Keeps well in a sealed container in the refrigerator for 2 to 3 weeks.

SUBS AND SWAPS: You can top this bark with any of your favorite toppings.

PER SERVING Calories: 567; Saturated Fat: 38g; Total Fat: 56g; Protein: 1g; Total Carbs: 11g; Fiber: 0g; Sodium: 236mg

Plantain Chocolate Nut Cookies

Prep time: 20 minutes · *Cook time:* 60 minutes · *Makes 10 cookies*

LOW FODMAP | VEGAN

A grain-free, whole-foods cookie full of potassium, fiber, polyphenols, healthy fats, nuts, seeds, and chocolate that tastes like a warm banana sundae? Don't mind if I do! These are a delicious and satisfying dessert alternative, relatively low in sugar, yet surprisingly decadent.

2 yellow plantains

1 cup almond flour

4 tablespoons arrowroot flour

1 tablespoon chia seeds

¼ teaspoon baking powder

¼ teaspoon baking soda

1 tablespoon apple cider vinegar

½ cup walnuts

½ cup shelled pumpkin seeds

1 cup bittersweet chocolate chips

1. Preheat the oven to 350°F. Line a baking sheet with parchment paper.

2. You don't need to peel plantains to cook them. Just cut into 4-inch segments and steam the plantains in a bowl set over a pot of boiling water for 8 to 10 minutes. Allow them to cool until they are safe to handle, then peel.

3. In a food processor, combine the plantains, almond and arrowroot flours, chia seeds, baking power and soda, vinegar, walnuts, and pumpkin seeds. Process until it forms a sticky dough, then mix in the chocolate chips by hand.

4. Separate the dough into 10 balls and spoon them onto the baking sheet, making sure to leave plenty of space around each one. Bake for 45 minutes, until the centers are soft but not gooey.

5. Cool on a wire rack to fully set.

SUBS AND SWAPS: If FODMAPs aren't your issue you can swap cooked sweet potato or winter squash for the plantains, and use any nuts you like—or no nuts at all. If you like raisins you can easily mix in ½ cup when you add the chocolate chips.

PER SERVING (1 COOKIE) Calories: 271; Saturated Fat: 6g; Total Fat: 19g; Protein: 6g; Total Carbs: 26g; Fiber: 4g; Sodium: 40mg

Mum's Flourless Chocolate Cake

Prep time: 10 minutes · *Cook time:* 25 minutes · *Serves:* 10

LOW FODMAP | VEGETARIAN

If you're going to eat chocolate cake, you might as well make it the richest kind around. This is my dear English mum's recipe, slightly altered to be dairy free. So simple yet so satisfying. All you need is a hot cuppa' (that's tea!) to make it a perfect treat.

½ cup coconut oil, plus extra for greasing

1 cup bittersweet chocolate chips

¾ cup coconut sugar

¼ teaspoon sea salt

1 teaspoon pure vanilla extract

½ cup unsweetened cocoa powder

3 eggs

1. Preheat the oven to 375°F. Grease an 8-inch round baking pan with a little extra coconut oil.

2. Heat some water in a pot over the stove on medium heat. When it starts to simmer, set a heatproof bowl on top of the pot and add the chocolate chips and coconut oil. Remove from heat immediately when they melt, so they don't get too hot. Transfer to a large mixing bowl.

3. Add the coconut sugar, salt, vanilla, and cocoa powder, and mix well. Add the eggs, whisking briefly between each one, until the batter is smooth.

4. Pour the batter into the prepared pan and bake for 20 to 25 minutes, making sure not to overbake. The cake is done when the top has formed a thin crust, and will solidify more as it cools.

SUBS AND SWAPS: If you can tolerate butter from grass-fed cows, it's delicious in place of the coconut oil.

PER SERVING Calories: 275; Saturated Fat: 14g; Total Fat: 20g; Protein: 4g; Total Carbs: 27g; Fiber: 3g; Sodium: 66mg

Harvest Moon Raspberry Balsamic Dressing, Page 141

CHAPTER 12

Dressings, Sauces, and Bone Broth

Green Herb Oil

Prep time: 5 minutes · *Makes 2 cups*

30 MINUTES | LOW FODMAP | NUT FREE | VEGAN

This is my favorite condiment to make every week. It's actually a great mayonnaise stand-in, protein topper, and an opportunity to add a burst of flavor and polyphenols to nearly any veggie dish. It's also an incredible way to get more herbs into your daily diet. Remember, herbs are our phytonutrient superheroes, so if you're aiming to eat more of these anti-inflammatories, then Green Herb Oil is going to be your new favorite too.

1 cup extra-virgin olive oil

2 cups fresh parsley, basil, or cilantro

¼ cup fresh fine herbs, such as thyme, oregano, rosemary, sage, mint leaves, and tarragon

¼ to ½ teaspoon sea salt

½ large lemon, juiced

1. Add your chosen ingredients to a blender or food processor and blend until smooth. You can put the larger herbs (cilantro, basil, parsley) in stems and all, while you'll need to pick the leaves off the fine herbs.

2. Taste for flavor and seasoning. If you want this as more of an herb sauce, add more oil. If you want a chunky spread, add more herbs.

PER SERVING (2 TABLESPOONS) Calories: 113; Saturated Fat: 2g; Total Fat: 13g; Protein: 0g; Total Carbs: 1g; Fiber: 1g; Sodium: 64mg

CULINARY IDEAS
Hawaiian pesto: 3 cups basil + ½ cup chopped macadamia nuts
Heavy metal detox: 3 cups cilantro
Minted spread: 2 cups parsley + 1 cup mint leaves
Chimichurri: 1 cup parsley + 2 tablespoons fresh oregano + 4 garlic cloves + 2 teaspoons crushed red pepper flakes + ¼ cup red wine vinegar

Harvest Moon Raspberry Balsamic Dressing

Prep time: 10 minutes · *Makes 1½ cups*

30 MINUTES | LOW FODMAP | NUT FREE | VEGAN

I'd only had low-fat balsamic dressing until I moved to Kaua'i and tasted what balsamic is supposed to taste like. Delicious! Real olive oil and tangy sweet balsamic, when blended with fresh raspberries, makes a luxurious salad dressing full of fresh antioxidants and flavor. It's so easy to make at home, do I seriously have no idea why I kept buying expensive, flavorless options.

½ cup extra-virgin olive oil

¼ cup balsamic vinegar

1 cup fresh raspberries, or frozen, then defrosted and drained

1 teaspoon Dijon mustard

¼ to ½ teaspoon sea salt

1. Put the oil, vinegar, raspberries, mustard, and salt in a blender or food processor, and blend until smooth.

2. Keeps well in the refrigerator in a glass jar for about 1 week.

SUBS AND SWAPS: Replace the raspberries with strawberries and a handful of basil, or blueberries and mint for something different.

POWER BOOST: Extra-virgin olive oil is made from cold-pressed olives, whereas regular olive oil blends different types of olive oils together for a refined, and less antioxidant-rich oil. That's why extra-virgin is your top choice for polyphenol content, vitamin E, and antioxidants. An at-home test for the purity of your olive oil: place it in the refrigerator. If it hardens, it's quite pure! If it stays very liquid-y, it's probably mixed with yucky oils.

PER SERVING (2 TABLESPOONS) Calories: 79; Saturated Fat: 1g; Total Fat: 9g; Protein: 0g; Total Carbs: 1g; Fiber: 1g; Sodium: 44mg

Fertility Goddess Dressing

Prep time: 10 minutes · *Makes about 1½ cups*

30 MINUTES | LOW FODMAP | NUT FREE | VEGAN

After 10 years as a strict vegan I ended up craving tahini on everything. Now I know it's because tahini is full of B vitamins, iron, zinc, and copper, nutrients often found more abundantly in animal products. My body was craving these nutrients! The sesame in tahini has been shown to improve the uptake of vitamin E, a nutrient essential for fertility and found abundantly in olive oil and avocados. Cheers to fertility!

½ cup tahini

½ cup extra-virgin olive oil

3 tablespoons coconut aminos

2 tablespoons apple cider vinegar

¼ teaspoon sea salt

⅛ teaspoon black pepper

1 ripe avocado

¼ cup filtered water (optional)

1. Put the tahini, oil, coconut aminos, vinegar, salt, pepper, and avocado in a blender or food processor, and blend until smooth.

2. If you prefer a thinner dressing, add filtered water to get the desired consistency.

3. Keeps well in the refrigerator in a glass jar for about 2 weeks.

POWER BOOST: Add 1 to 2 tablespoons of Green Herb Oil (page 140) for an herbed dressing, which will significantly raise the polyphenols and make this dressing extra anti-inflammatory.

PER SERVING (2 TABLESPOONS) Calories: 161; Saturated Fat: 2g; Total Fat: 16g; Protein: 2g; Total Carbs: 4g; Fiber: 2g; Sodium: 57mg

Fermented Ketchupepper

Prep time: 10 minutes · *Ferment time:* 2 to 3 days · *Makes 1 quart*

NUT FREE | VEGAN

Before the age of refrigeration, or even canning, everything preserved was fermented. Think about that: A whole winter without refrigerators or even airtight jars meant you really relied on probiotic bacteria to keep your food from spoiling. Ketchup was no different, and although the recipe has changed over the centuries, you and your gut can enjoy it in its probiotic state with this fun and easy kitchen experiment.

1 bottle organic ketchup

1 cup roasted red peppers

2 tablespoons sugar-free sriracha or other hot sauce

¼ teaspoon garlic powder

1 teaspoon apple cider vinegar

4 lactobacillus-based probiotic pills or ½ cup brine from your Fermented Shreds (page 124)

1. Put the ketchup, peppers, sriracha, garlic powder, vinegar, and probiotic pills in a blender or food processor and blend until smooth.

2. Pour into a sterile jar, and loosely cover with a lid so it can breathe. Leave on the counter for 2 to 3 days to ferment. The sweet flavor should be replaced with a vinegar-like flavor.

3. When it tastes right to you, screw on the lid and move to the refrigerator. It keeps well for 4 to 6 months.

SUBS AND SWAPS: If you want to start easily, just mix the store-bought ketchup with the probiotic pills for a simple fermented ketchup. Play around with seasonings from there, adding chiles and honey for a sweet chili sauce, or adding molasses and cloves for a pseudo-barbecue sauce.

LOW FODMAP: You'll have to find a FODMAP-friendly ketchup, such as one sold by Fody Foods, and omit the garlic powder.

PER SERVING (¼ CUP) Calories: 57; Saturated Fat: 0g; Total Fat: 1g; Protein: 0g; Total Carbs: 9g; Fiber: 0g; Sodium: 454mg

Fermented Coco-Kefir or Coconut Sour Cream

Prep time: 2 minutes · *Ferment time:* 2 to 3 days · *Makes 1½ cups*

LOW FODMAP | NUT FREE | VEGAN

Making your own coconut ferments is fun, easy, and a better option than some varieties of pricey coconut products that have a slew of nasty ingredients in them. Plus, I've never seen coconut sour cream on the market, so your dairy-free friends will beg you for the recipe. I like to ferment 2 to 3 cans every Thursday night, so I have them ready by Sunday for the coming week.

1 (12-ounce) can full-fat coconut milk for coco-kefir, or 1 (12-ounce) can heavy coconut cream for sour cream

3 lactobacillus-based probiotic pills

1. Pour the coconut milk into a sterile glass jar, add the probiotic pills, tightly screw on the lid, and shake, shake, shake.

2. Lightly unscrew the lid so the contents can breathe, and leave on the counter for 2 to 3 days. The longer you wait, the more sour it will be.

3. Taste after 2 days. When it's the way you like, screw on the lid and place in the refrigerator. This will keep in the refrigerator for 1 week or more.

SUBS AND SWAPS: If you can't find canned heavy coconut cream for the sour cream, you can ferment a regular can of coconut milk and, when finished, place in the refrigerator to chill. As it does so, the cream will rise to the top. Scoop it off and this will be your sour cream.

PER SERVING (2 TABLESPOONS) Calories: 65; Saturated Fat: 6g; Total Fat: 8g; Protein: 1g; Total Carbs: 2g; Fiber: 1g; Sodium: 4mg

Cashew Cheese

Prep time: 10 minutes · *Makes about 2½ cups*

30 MINUTES | VEGAN

Cashew cheese is a gift from heaven for any dairy lovers out there suddenly unable to eat cheese. This was me until I discovered the power of the cashew. Creamy and rich in healthy fats and proteins, it's a great cheese stand-in as a topping, spread, or dip. You can also make it as thick or as runny as you want, depending on how you plan to use it.

2 cup cashews, soaked in 4 cups water for at least 3 hours and drained

3 tablespoons coconut aminos

¼ cup nutritional yeast

1 tablespoon apple cider vinegar

¼ teaspoon sea salt

½ teaspoon Dijon mustard

¼ teaspoon garlic powder

½ red bell pepper, seeded and roughly chopped

1. Put the cashews, coconut aminos, nutritional yeast, vinegar, salt, mustard, garlic powder, and bell pepper in a blender or food processor and blend until smooth.

2. If you prefer a thinner dressing, add filtered water to the desired consistency.

3. Keeps well in a glass jar in the refrigerator for 3 to 4 days.

POWER BOOST: Add 1 to 2 tablespoons Green Herb Oil (page 140) for an herbed dressing, which will raise the polyphenol content to make this extra anti-inflammatory.

LOW FODMAP: Leave out the garlic powder, and substitute macadamia nuts for cashews. They may not blend as fully as cashews, but the flavor is still there, and utterly satisfying.

PER SERVING (2 TABLESPOONS) Calories: 86; Saturated Fat: 1g; Total Fat: 6g; Protein: 4g; Total Carbs: 6g; Fiber: 1g; Sodium: 31mg

Almond Satay Sauce

Prep time: 5 minutes · *Makes about 1½ cups*

30 MINUTES | VEGAN

Foregoing peanuts isn't hard when you replace them with creamy vitamin E–, mineral-, and antioxidant-rich almonds. I love to have this awesome alternative to a peanut sauce in the refrigerator at all times to pour on a stir-fry, on a wrap, or as a dip for some fresh farmers' market veggies. Try it with other nut butters, too.

½ cup organic almond butter

⅛ to ¼ cup fresh lime juice

¼ cup coconut aminos

¼ teaspoon sea salt

1 teaspoon rice vinegar

1 teaspoon red pepper flakes

½ teaspoon garlic powder

½ cup full-fat coconut milk

1. Put the almond butter, lime juice, coconut aminos, salt, vinegar, red pepper flakes, garlic powder, and coconut milk into a blender or food processor, and blend until smooth.

2. This will keep in a glass jar in the refrigerator for up to 1 week.

LEFTOVERS AND EXTRAS: If you love this sauce, double or triple the recipe and freeze the leftovers. It's so simple to make, and you'll save lots of time on prep and clean up.

LOW FODMAP: Leave out the garlic powder.

PER SERVING (2 TABLESPOONS) Calories: 41; Saturated Fat: 3g; Total Fat: 3g; Protein: 1g; Total Carbs: 3g; Fiber: 0g; Sodium: 56mg

Ohana Hawaiian Stir-Fry Sauce

Prep time: 5 minutes · *Makes about 1 cup*

30 MINUTES | VEGAN

When you give up soy, gluten, and sugar, you also give up many of your usual condiments like teriyaki, barbecue sauce, and other favorites. Don't worry! I've got you covered with my own family recipe I know your family will love as well. You should never have to skimp on flavor when transitioning to a whole-foods lifestyle, nor should your family.

1½ teaspoons apple cider vinegar

3 garlic cloves

2 tablespoons Chinese five-spice powder

1 teaspoon red pepper flakes

¼ cup plus 2 tablespoons unsweetened pineapple juice

½ cup coconut aminos

1. Put the vinegar, garlic, five-spice powder, red pepper flakes, pineapple juice, and coconut aminos into a blender and blend until smooth.

2. Taste for flavor, knowing the red pepper flakes will slightly intensify with heat as it cooks.

3. Keep in a glass jar in the refrigerator for up to 1 week.

SUBS AND SWAPS: You can use lemon or lime juice instead of pineapple juice if you prefer a lower sugar option. But you can't substitute out the five-spice powder; it's a crucial ingredient, so make sure to stock it in your pantry.

LOW FODMAP: Leave out the garlic.

PER SERVING (2 TABLESPOONS) Calories: 30; Saturated Fat: 0g; Total Fat: 0g; Protein: 2g; Total Carbs: 5g; Fiber: 1g; Sodium: 17mg

Bone Broth

Prep time: 20 minutes · *Cook time:* 4 to 24 hours · *Makes ½ gallon*

Bone broth has become trendy, but with good reason. This slow-simmered broth offers pre-digested amino acids for those of us with severely compromised digestion, and is über rich in glycine, an amino acid that regulates inflammation in the body. When we're deficient we can develop chronic inflammation, and that's why bone broth is especially essential for women with endometriosis.

A pot worth of collagen-rich bones, such as

6 knuckle bones

1 carrot, barely chopped

1 onion, barely chopped

Filtered water

Sea salt

Apple cider vinegar

1. Roast the bones in the oven first—this adds yummy flavor! Place on a baking sheet and broil on high, about 10 minutes per side.

2. Add the bones to a large pot with the carrot and onion (or any veggies), and add enough filtered water to just cover the bones. Add a spoonful of salt, a dash vinegar, and barely simmer on very low heat for 24 hours if you're cooking on the stovetop or using a slow cooker.

3. If you're using an Instant Pot® electric pressure cooker, cook on high pressure for 4 hours (which is why having an Instant Pot® is very helpful if you make lots of broth, which I recommend).

SUBS AND SWAPS: As you can see, the amount of ingredients here isn't very important. You can make bone broth with one bone or 10 bones; chicken, lamb, or any other bone; no veggies or a lot of veggies. The important thing is your ratio of bones to water. When you're making broth, simply *just* cover the bones with water and simmer. If you use too much water, your broth won't gel, nor have much flavor.

POWER BOOST: To make this more anti-inflammatory, I love to make a Thai-inspired broth with lemongrass, garlic, ginger, kaffir lime leaf, and turmeric.

LOW FODMAP: Leave out the onion.

PER SERVING (1 CUP) Calories: 64; Saturated Fat: 2g; Total Fat: 4g; Protein: 6g; Total Carbs: 1g; Fiber: 0g; Sodium: 109mg

SYMPTOM TRACKER

WEEK ONE

Use the following tables to track your symptoms throughout the month with the emphasis on observing rather than solving. When we're mindful and observe what's happening and when, it can help us see potential reasons or timing behind some of our most perplexing symptoms.

Dates (M/D/Y – M/D/Y): _____

	S	M	T	W	TH	F	S
ENERGY: 1 = low 10 = high							
PAIN: 1 = low 10 = high							
STRESS LEVELS: 1 = low 10 = high							
DAY OF CYCLE (first day of period is day 1)							
NOTABLE SYMPTOMS (circle those which apply)	Bloating Nausea Indigestion Headache Insomnia Cravings Allergies	Bloating Nausea Indigestion Headache Insomnia Cravings Allergies	Bloating Nausea Indigestion Headache Insomnia Cravings Allergies	Bloating Nausea Indigestion Headache Insomnia Cravings Allergies	Bloating Nausea Indigestion Headache Insomnia Cravings Allergies	Bloating Nausea Indigestion Headache Insomnia Cravings Allergies	Bloating Nausea Indigestion Headache Insomnia Cravings Allergies

WEEK TWO

Dates (M/D/Y - M/D/Y): _____

	S	M	T	W	TH	F	S
ENERGY: 1 = low 10 = high							
PAIN: 1 = low 10 = high							
STRESS LEVELS: 1 = low 10 = high							
DAY OF CYCLE (first day of period is day 1)							
NOTABLE SYMPTOMS (circle those which apply)	Bloating Nausea Indigestion Headache Insomnia Cravings Allergies	Bloating Nausea Indigestion Headache Insomnia Cravings Allergies	Bloating Nausea Indigestion Headache Insomnia Cravings Allergies	Bloating Nausea Indigestion Headache Insomnia Cravings Allergies	Bloating Nausea Indigestion Headache Insomnia Cravings Allergies	Bloating Nausea Indigestion Headache Insomnia Cravings Allergies	Bloating Nausea Indigestion Headache Insomnia Cravings Allergies

WEEK THREE

Dates (*M/D/Y – M/D/Y*): _____

	S	M	T	W	TH	F	S
ENERGY: 1 = low 10 = high							
PAIN: 1 = low 10 = high							
STRESS LEVELS: 1 = low 10 = high							
DAY OF CYCLE (first day of period is day 1)							
NOTABLE SYMPTOMS (circle those which apply)	Bloating Nausea Indigestion Headache Insomnia Cravings Allergies	Bloating Nausea Indigestion Headache Insomnia Cravings Allergies	Bloating Nausea Indigestion Headache Insomnia Cravings Allergies	Bloating Nausea Indigestion Headache Insomnia Cravings Allergies	Bloating Nausea Indigestion Headache Insomnia Cravings Allergies	Bloating Nausea Indigestion Headache Insomnia Cravings Allergies	Bloating Nausea Indigestion Headache Insomnia Cravings Allergies

WEEK FOUR

Dates (M/D/Y – M/D/Y): _____

	S	M	T	W	TH	F	S
ENERGY: 1 = low 10 = high							
PAIN: 1 = low 10 = high							
STRESS LEVELS: 1 = low 10 = high							
DAY OF CYCLE (first day of period is day 1)							
NOTABLE SYMPTOMS (circle those which apply)	Bloating Nausea Indigestion Headache Insomnia Cravings Allergies	Bloating Nausea Indigestion Headache Insomnia Cravings Allergies	Bloating Nausea Indigestion Headache Insomnia Cravings Allergies	Bloating Nausea Indigestion Headache Insomnia Cravings Allergies	Bloating Nausea Indigestion Headache Insomnia Cravings Allergies	Bloating Nausea Indigestion Headache Insomnia Cravings Allergies	Bloating Nausea Indigestion Headache Insomnia Cravings Allergies

THE DIRTY DOZEN™ AND THE CLEAN FIFTEEN™

Each year, the Environmental Working Group compiles a list of the best and worst pesticide loads found in commercial crops. The list is updated annually, and you can find it online at EWG.org/FoodNews. The Dirty Dozen™ are foods that have high levels of pesticide residues when conventionally grown.

- strawberries
- spinach
- kale
- nectarines
- apples
- grapes
- peaches
- cherries
- pears
- tomatoes
- celery
- potatoes

The Clean Fifteen™ were found to have the lowest amounts of pesticide contamination in 2014, and are considered safe to buy conventionally grown (nonorganic):

- avocados
- sweet corn
- pineapples
- sweet peas (frozen)
- onions
- papayas
- eggplants
- asparagus
- kiwis
- cabbages
- cauliflower
- cantaloupes
- broccoli
- mushrooms
- honeydew melons

MEASUREMENTS AND CONVERSIONS

VOLUME EQUIVALENTS (LIQUID)

US STANDARD	US STANDARD (OUNCES)	METRIC (APPROXIMATE)
2 tablespoons	1 fl. oz.	30 mL
¼ cup	2 fl. oz.	60 mL
½ cup	4 fl. oz.	120 mL
1 cup	8 fl. oz.	240 mL
1½ cups	12 fl. oz.	355 mL
2 cups or 1 pint	16 fl. oz.	475 mL
4 cups or 1 quart	32 fl. oz.	1 L
1 gallon	128 fl. oz.	4 L

OVEN TEMPERATURES

FAHRENHEIT	CELSIUS (APPROXIMATE)
250°F	120°C
300°F	150°C
325°F	165°C
350°F	180°C
375°F	190°C
400°F	200°C
425°F	220°C
450°F	230°C

VOLUME EQUIVALENTS (DRY)

US STANDARD	METRIC (APPROXIMATE)
⅛ teaspoon	0.5 mL
¼ teaspoon	1 mL
½ teaspoon	2 mL
¾ teaspoon	4 mL
1 teaspoon	5 mL
1 tablespoon	15 mL
¼ cup	59 mL
⅓ cup	79 mL
½ cup	118 mL
⅔ cup	156 mL
¾ cup	177 mL
1 cup	235 mL
2 cups or 1 pint	475 mL
3 cups	700 mL
4 cups or 1 quart	1 L

WEIGHT EQUIVALENTS

US STANDARD	METRIC (APPROXIMATE)
½ ounce	15 g
1 ounce	30 g
2 ounces	60 g
4 ounces	115 g
8 ounces	225 g
12 ounces	340 g
16 ounces or 1 pound	455 g

RESOURCES

ENDOMETRIOSIS AND TREATMENT

www.HealEndo.com

My personal site about endometriosis and holistic healing. Here you can dive deep into many facets of nutrition, endo-belly, natural movement, alignment, detoxing, and learning to live again.

www.EndoFound.org

The website of the Endometriosis Foundation of America, an *incredible* resource for everything about endometriosis. Here you can learn about surgery, advocacy, and how to give back.

www.EndoWhat.com

An incredible documentary on endo, surgery, treatment, advocacy, and beyond.

NUTRITION, DIET, AND STRESS

AutoImmuneWellness.com

This site is dedicated to everything about the Paleo Autoimmune Protocol (AIP) gut-healing diet and the link to diet and autoimmune diseases.

www.MonashFODMAP.com

This up-to-date site (research in this realm is constantly updated) from Monash University lists high-FODMAP foods.

FodyFoods.com

Fody Foods is America's first low-FODMAP food and condiment company.

Calm.com

The Calm App, meditation techniques that help you relax slowly but surely.

BOOKS

Ballantyne, Sarah. *The Paleo Approach*. Las Vegas: Victory Belt Publishing Inc., 2013.

Katz, Sandor. *The Art of Fermentation*. White River Junction, Vermont: Chelsea Green Publishing, 2012.

Nichols, Lily. *Real Food for Pregnancy*. n.p.: Lily Nichols, 2018.

Norman, Abby. *Ask Me About My Uterus*. New York: Bold Type Books, 2018.

Seckin, Tamer. *The Doctor Will See You Now*. Nashville: Turner Publishing Company, 2016.

Shanahan, Catherine. *Deep Nutrition*. New York: Flatiron Books, 2008.

REFERENCES

Anastasi, Emanuela, et al. "Low Levels of 25-OH Vitamin D in Women with Endometriosis and Associated Pelvic Pain." *Clinical Chemistry and Laboratory Medicine* 55, no. 12 (April 2017): e282–e284. doi: 10.1515/cclm-2017-0016.

Ata, Baris, et al. "The Endobiota Study: Comparison of Vaginal, Cervical and Gut Microbiota Between Women with Stage 3/4 Endometriosis and Healthy Controls." *Scientific Reports* 9, no. 2204 (February 2019). doi: 10.1038/s41598-019-39700-6.

Bailey, Michael, and Christopher L. Coe, "Endometriosis is Associated with an Altered Profile of Intestinal Microflora in Female Rhesus Monkeys." *Human Reproduction* 17, no. 7 (July 2002): 1704–1708. doi: 10.1093/humrep/17.7.1704.

Bernardo, D., et al. "Is Gliadin Really Safe for Non-Coeliac Individuals? Production of Interleukin 15 in Biopsy Culture from Non-Coeliac Individuals Challenged with Gliadin Peptides." *Gut* 56, no. 6 (June 2007): 889–890. doi: 10.1136/gut.2006 .118265.

Bulletti, C., M.E. Coccia, S. Battistoni, et al. "Endometriosis and Infertility." *Journal of Assisted Reproduction and Genetics* 27, no. 8 (2010): 441–447. doi: 10.1007/ s10815-010-9436-1.

Cuevas, Marielly, et al. "Stress Exacerbates Endometriosis Manifestations and Inflammatory Parameters in an Animal Model." *Reproductive Sciences* 19, no. 8 (August 2012): 851–862. doi: 10.1177/1933719112438443.

Dmitrovic, Romana. "Transvaginal Color Doppler Study of Uterine Blood Flow in Primary Dysmenorrhea." *Acta Obstetricia et Gynecologica Scandinavica* 79, no. 12 (December 2000): 1112–1116. doi: 10.1080/00016340009169273.

Erten, Ozlem Ulas, et al. "Vitamin C is Effective for the Prevention and Regression of Endometriotic Implants in an Experimentally Induced Rat Model of Endometriosis." *Taiwanese Journal of Obstetrics and Gynecology* 55, no. 2 (April 2016): 251–257. doi: 10.1016/j.tjog.2015.07.004.

Etxeberria, Usune, Alfredo Fernández-Quintela, Fermín I. Milagro, Leixuri Aguirre, J. Alfredo Martínez, and María P. Portillo. "Impact of Polyphenols and Polyphenol-Rich Dietary Sources on Gut Microbiota Composition." *Journal of Agricultural and Food Chemistry* 61, no. 40 (October 2013): 9517–9533. doi: 10.1021/jf402506c.

Evensen, Nikki, and Phyllis Braun. "The Effects of Tea Polyphenols on Candida Albicans: Inhibition of Biofilm Formation and Proteasome Inactivation." *Canadian Journal of Microbiology* 55, no. 9 (2009): 1033–1039. doi: 10.1139/W09-058.

Halpern, Gabriela, Eduardo Schor, and Alexander Kopelman. "Nutritional Aspects Related to Endometriosis." *Revista da Associação Médica Brasileira* 61, no. 6 (November/December 2015). doi: 10.1590/1806-9282.61.06.519.

Herington, Jennifer, et al. "Dietary Fish Oil Supplementation Inhibits Formation of Endometriosis-Associated Adhesions in a Chimeric Mouse Model." *Fertility and Sterility* 99, no. 2 (2013): 543–550. doi: 10.1016/j.fertnstert.2012.10.007.

Khan, K.N., et al. "17β-estradiol and Lipopolysaccharide Additively Promote Pelvic Inflammation and Growth of Endometriosis." *Reproductive Sciences* 22, no. 5 (2015): 585–594. doi: 10.1177/1933719114556487.

Khan, K.N., et al. "Bacterial Contamination Hypothesis: A New Concept in Endometriosis." *Reproductive Medicine and Biology* 17, no. 2 (January 2018): 125–133. doi: 10.1002/rmb2.12083.

Laschke, Matthias, and Michael Menger. "The Gut Microbiota: A Puppet Master in the Pathogenesis of Endometriosis?" *American Journal of Obstetrics and Gynecology* 215, no. 1 (July 2016): 68.e1–68.e4. doi: 10.1016/j.ajog.2016.02.036.

Levine, Hagai, et al. "Temporal Trends in Sperm Count: A Systematic Review and Meta-Regression Analysis." *Human Reproduction Update* 23, no. 6 (November/December 2017): 646–659. doi: 10.1093/humupd/dmx022.

Lin, Henry C. "Small Intestinal Bacterial Overgrowth: A Framework for Understanding Irritable Bowel Syndrome." *JAMA* 292, no. 7 (2004): 852–858. doi: 10.1001/jama.292.7.852.

Maroun, P., et al. "Relevance of Gastrointestinal Symptoms in Endometriosis." *ANZJOG* 49, no. 4 (July 2009): 411–414. doi: 10.1111/j.1479-828X .2009.01030.x.

Marziali, M., et al. "Gluten-Free Diet: A New Strategy for Management of Painful Endometriosis Related Symptoms?" *Edizioni Minerva Medica* 67, no. 6 (December 2012): 499–504.

Mathias, J.R., et al. "Relation of Endometriosis and Neuromuscular Disease of the Gastrointestinal Tract: New Insights." *Fertility and Sterility* 70, no. 1 (July 1998): 81–88. doi: 10.1016/S0015-0282(98)00096-X.

Messalli, E.M., et al. "The Possible Role of Zinc in the Etiopathogenesis of Endometriosis." *Clinical and Experimental Obstetrics and Gynecology* 41, no. 5 (2014): 541–546.

McIntosh, Keith, D.E. Reed, T. Schneider, et al. "FODMAPs Alter Symptoms and the Metabolome of Patients with IBS: a Randomised Controlled Trial." *Gut* 66, no. 7 (July 2017):1241–1251. doi: 10.1136/gutjnl-2015-311339.

Mier-Cabrera, Jennifer, et al. "Women with Endometriosis Improved Their Peripheral Antioxidant Markers After the Application of a High Antioxidant Diet." *Reproductive Biology and Endocrinology* 7, no. 54 (May 2009). doi: 10.1186/1477-7827-7-54.

Pavone, M.E., et al. "Endometriosis Expresses a Molecular Pattern Consistent with Decreased Retinoid Uptake, Metabolism and Action." *Human Reproduction* 26, no. 8 (August 2011): 2157–2164. doi: 10.1093/humrep/der172.

Santanam, Nalini, et al. "Antioxidant Supplementation Reduces Endometriosis-Related Pelvic Pain in Humans." *Translational Research* 161, no. 3 (March 2013):189–195. doi: 10.1016/j.trsl.2012.05.001.

Seeber, Beata, et al. "The Vitamin E-Binding Protein Afamin is Altered Significantly in the Peritoneal Fluid of Women with Endometriosis." *Fertility and Sterility* 94, no. 7 (2010): 2923–2926. doi: 10.1016/j.fertnstert.2010.05.008.

Zhao, R.H., W.W. Sun, Y. Liu, et al. "Chinese Medicine in Management of Chronic Disease Endometriosis." *Chinese Journal of Integrative Medicine* (January 2018). doi: 10.1007/s11655-018-2937-3.

RECIPE LABEL INDEX

INDEX

ACKNOWLEDGMENTS

Having endometriosis isn't easy, which is why I first and foremost thank my husband, Mason, for always believing in me, for never being embarrassed about my "female" issues, and for never faltering in your support. I honestly wouldn't be where I am today without you. You are my soulmate; my rock.

Thanks to my incredibly supportive and loving parents, Marion and Ron, and to my brother, Josh, who taught me to be resilient in the face of challenges. You gave me the tools I needed to climb mountains, even the toughest ones.

I'm so grateful to my extended family, my mother-in-law, Harvest, who inspired my health and healing journey more than she knows. To my best friends—what amazing women you all are. And of course, thanks to my son, Elias, who is living proof that miracles do happen.

ABOUT THE AUTHOR

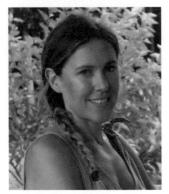

Katie Edmonds is a Nutritional Therapy Consultant (NTC) certified through the Nutritional Therapy Association, and a Paleo Autoimmune Protocol (AIP) certified coach. Her free educational website, HealEndo.com, has attracted tens of thousands of women seeking solutions, while she helps clients one-on-one through her online practice. As a staunch advocate of understanding endometriosis as a whole-body disease, she wrote the book on endo-belly, connecting the severity of endometriosis to gut health, and is passionate about helping women get the care they truly need to recover their lives. She lives on the north shore of Kaua'i.